COMMUNICATION AND PRESE SKILLS FOR HEALTHCARE PROFESSIONALS

- A Simple Guide

DR SYED RAZA

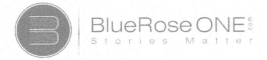
BlueRose ONE
Stories Matter

First Published in April 2023

ISBN: 978-93-5741-578-1

BLUEROSE PUBLISHERS
www.BlueRoseONE.com
info@bluerosepublishers.com
+91 8882 898 898

Cover Design:
Tahira Akhtar

Typographic Design:
Namrata Saini

Distributed by: BlueRose, Amazon, Flipkart

Contents

COMMUNICATION SKILLS IN HEALTHCARE

Chapter 1: Introduction to communication and presentation skills in healthcare 3

Chapter 2: Tools for health communication.. 27

Chapter 3: Why communication in healthcare is important?.. 42

Chapter 4: How to communicate effectively in healthcare? 60

Chapter 5: Ethical and legal aspects of communication in healthcare 76

PRESENTATION SKILLS IN HEALTHCARE

Chapter 6: Delivering a great presentation in healthcare - Tips and Tricks 95

Chapter 7: Preparations before your presentation 104

Chapter 8: Do's and Dont's during a presentation 120

Chapter 9: After your presentation – Reflection and Feedback 135

Chapter 10: Your professional journey as a powerful communicator and presenter 155

Conclusion.. 162

COMMUNICATION SKILLS IN HEALTHCARE

CHAPTER 1

Introduction to communication and presentation skills in healthcare

"The two words 'information' and 'communication' are often used interchangeably, but they signify quite different things. Information is giving out; communication is getting through". -Sydney J. Harris

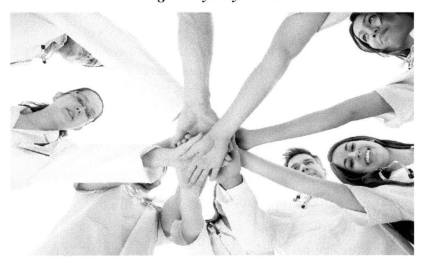

Communication - reaching out

Communication: what, why, where and how?

The word ***communication*** originates from the Latin word, ***communicare*** which came from ***communis***, meaning ***"common"***. The word, first used in 1529, is interpreted by Merriam-Webster Dictionary as

"to convey knowledge or information: make known."

According to this definition, the word ***"communication"*** not only implies the sharing of information, but also being certain that the information has made the necessary impact it was meant to make: ***getting through.***

Ever since the humankind has inhabited the earth, the need for communication has only grown. It was for the need of communication that different languages were invented and developed. Wanting to be heard and understood is one of the basic needs of anyone's personal and social life. Communication, through language, formed the key for the early man to *"identify"* himself as a part of certain *"group"*, to travel, to settle, to thrive, to form *"bonds"*, to reproduce, to envy, to fight, to win, to be proud of: everything needs communication. After all, isn't one's language something to be proud of?

It is predictable that the need to influence and connect with others are among the most important reasons for the emergence of early forms of writing. This need is also evident in many other forms of communication that seek to create feelings of approval, recognition, or friendliness, among others.

Let's look at it from another perspective. What is the first biggest achievement of an infant during the first or second year of his life in terms of social aspect of his development? No doubt, it's the infant's effort to communicate with the world around him for the first time – a baby's first words. Parents often agree that they make the first, real bond with the baby, or feel that *"connection"* only when the baby starts talking. Even when he just tries to respond with gestures, he is trying to communicate. In other words, *"expressions"* are also effective tools of communication.

So the essence of the word communication can be summarized as:

1. Exchange of information, between people by means of speaking, writing, language, common signs of expression and behaviors
2. A spoken or written message
3. An act of communicating
4. Rapport: a sense of mutual understanding and sympathy
5. A means of access or communication, just like *a connecting door*

Only through the deep reflection on the literal meaning of this word, communication, will we be able to understand the theory and practice of "health communication"

In fact, all of these meanings can relate to the modalities of health communication programs. As commonly with other forms of communication, health communication is ideally based on *two-way exchange of information* that uses a *"system of signs and behaviors understood by everyone involved."* This should be *accessible* and create *"mutual feelings of understanding, empathy and sympathy"* amongst members communicating with each other e.g. presenter and audience, health team and patients. Lastly, there must exist the *"communication channels"* (the way the communicator reaches the target audiences with a message e.g. health communication messages, materials, etc.). Do not forget that messages are the *"connecting doors"* that allow information to reach the audience by communication.

Health Communication – introduction:

The Centers for Disease Control and Prevention (CDC) define health communication as

"the study and use of communication strategies to inform and influence individual and community decisions that enhance health"

Health communications aims to influence individuals and communities. Health communication improves health outcomes by sharing the right *"health-related information"* with the patients in particular and community in general.

The word *influence* is also included in another definition of health communication as *"the art and technique of informing, affecting, and motivating individual, institutional, and public audiences about important health issues"* (U.S. Department of Health and Human Services, 2005)

Communication also creates a receptive, conducive and favorable environment in which information can be transmitted, comprehended, absorbed, and discussed by the intended audiences. An in-depth understanding of the basic needs, beliefs, taboos, behaviors, attitudes, lifestyle, and social customs are required. Communication's purpose is to share easily understandable messages. As Pearson and Nelson in 1991 termed it as *"a process of understanding and sharing meanings."*

If you can imagine a very easy to understand and practical implementation of this definition: cracking an innocent *joke* about personality trait of a *close friend* and a *colleague's/recent acquaintance's*. What do you reckon the difference in reactions would be? The friend would most probably laugh at the joke, while the colleague/recent acquaintance might get offended. In short, the magnitude of communication efforts is dependent on familiarity with the target audience. It is more likely for meanings to be shared and understood in the way communicators were intending them to be. Therefore, health communication, i.e. the communication in matters of life-and-death, is a long strategic process. It needs a true understanding of target audiences as well as the communicator's ability to adapt to them. A communicator redefines his communication goals, strategies, and activities on the basis of audience feedback.

Nonprofit organizations, public, private and commercial sectors have been using interventions in health communication successfully. According to World Health Organization, health communication in its true sense, is a multidisciplinary approach - it draws from numerous disciplines:

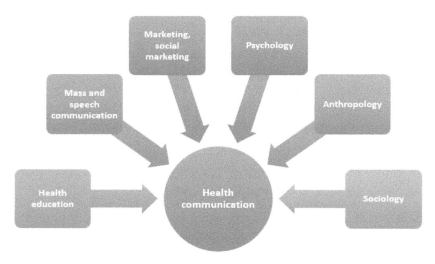

Health Communication as a multidisciplinary approach

Health communication is reliant on different communication activities, including *interpersonal communications, public relations, public advocacy, community mobilization, and professional communications.*

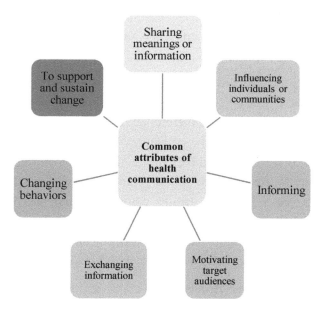

Common attributes of health communication

Successful health communication programs or campaigns always include **two** key elements:

- Long-term sustainability of the program
- Development of tools and steps of communication

They help in helping individuals and communities to adopt and maintain recommended behaviors, practices or policy changes. If we merge this practice-based perspective with many of the other definitions of health communication, a new and improved definition would look like this:

"Health communication is a multifaceted and multidisciplinary approach to reach different audiences and share health-related information with the goal of influencing, engaging, and supporting individuals, communities, health professionals, special groups, policymakers and the public to champion, introduce, adopt, or sustain a behavior, practice, or policy that will ultimately improve health outcomes"

Health communication is a dynamic, rapidly-evolving and prominent field in both public, nonprofit and commercial health sectors. Health communication can play a pivotal role to influence and support individuals, communities, health professionals and policymakers to adopt and implement behavioral practices and social/policy change that will lead to improved health outcomes.

Understanding health communication and its implementation

Having a solid understanding of health communication allows healthcare managers and professionals to identify training needs of staff and other health team members. It helps the organizations to create the right mind-set and capability that leads to successful use of communication approaches to reach specific goals of the target population

Health communication in the modern era

"Health communication is the use of communication techniques and modern age technologies to (positively) influence individuals, populations, and organizations for the purpose of promoting conditions conducive to human and environmental health"

(Maibach and Holtgrave, 2006).

Health communication is all about improving health outcomes by motivating people to modify behavior and social customs. It is a comprehensive approach that relies on the full understanding and involvement of its target audiences.

Health communication and its theoretical basis, both have evolved rapidly in the past four to five decades, which today, draws on a number of additional disciplines. Communicators are no longer treated just like those *"who write press releases"* but as *"fundamental members of the public health teams"*.

Communication is no longer considered a skill but a science – requiring mentoring and passion. It relies on the use of *vehicles* or *tools* (materials, activities, events, etc. to deliver a message through communication channels). Practitioners of health communication have always been trained "on-the-job." People from many different fields have been encouraged to enter health communication programs to meet human resource needs, including *demography, sociology, public health, psychology,* and different fields like *filmmaking, journalism and advertising* – all working together in a team.

In the mid-90s, owing to the increasing demand, schools all over the world started their own curricular programs in Health Communication which helped bring academic's attention to this emerging field. The number of publications rose, and the training moved to **"pre-service"** from **"in-service"**. The more technically competent the health educators are, the better the health outcomes will be. Health communication needs structured planning with perfect execution and fierce evaluation – possible only with adequate training. It is a lifetime learning endeavor and requires new training initiatives and tools. Beginning of this training should be academic setting but complemented by practical experience, observations, in-service training and continuing professional education.

The highest potential of health communication lies within a team effort. Finally, it is important to remember that there is no magic bullet that can address health issues. Health communication is a rapidly-evolving discipline and should seek help from evaluation. It should, from time to time, absorb the lessons and incorporate the changes based on them, through multidisciplinary interventions. This is indeed the essence and purpose of the "evaluation cycle".

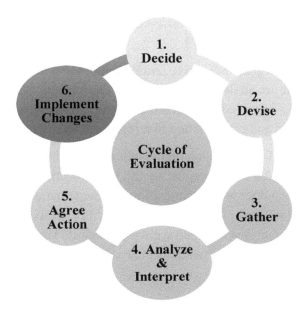

Cycle of evaluation

Key strategies of health communication:

There are several health communication approaches or strategies that can be followed to attain the ultimate goal of "better health outcomes":

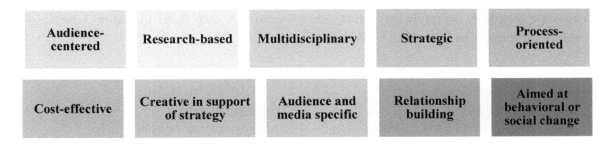

Let us discuss each strategy one by one.

1. <u>Patient-centered health communication</u>

Health communication is a long process that ultimately ends with the audience's wishes and fulfillment of their needs – better health outcomes. It could mean reduced recovery time, less hospital admissions, short stays in the hospital, better compliance to precautionary and therapeutic measures, etc.

The patients are not only "targets" but active participant in the whole "health communication" process where health issue are analyzed and culturally appropriate, cost-effective solutions are worked out. Patients are involved in researching and implementing chief strategies and activities. For this, patients and organization that represent them need to work together.

Let us take an example of a health communication program that is aiming to approach survivors of breast cancer. All the strategies should be planned, designed, shared, discussed, tested, and implemented together with organizations, patients/patient groups, team leaders and community representatives/local population. It is only fair to include patients and general population – they need to feel invested and well-represented. They are the *"protagonists"* of the action-plan that will bring about a behavioral or social change.

2. Research Based

Research provides the ground for successful health communication programs with assistance from good understanding of patients and their situations. This involves all the current programs as well as previous programs. In addition, it includes information learned about previous policies, social customs, hurdles and problems in addressing a specific health problem. The environment in which humans live affects their behavior. Creation of a receptive environment is mandatory which encourages the patients/community to discuss a health issues and support the "changes" that need to be made (by patients, their family members and their healthcare team). A comprehensive research program can help fulfil this aim. Traditional research techniques include these fundamental steps:

Draw situation analysis
• Analysis of an individual, the society, policies and behaviors that affect attitudes, social norms and policies concerning a health issue.

Development of profile
• Patient's/population's profile which includes a comprehensive, research-based description of their characteristics, demographics, essential requirements, social values, and attitudes.

Traditional research techniques

3. Multidisciplinary

The nature of health communication is *transdisciplinary* as it draws on multiple health disciplines and it recognizes the complexity of attaining *"psychosocial change."* This multifaceted approach stems from several practices and theories e.g. **health education, social marketing, theories of behavioral and social change theories**. Both private and commercial sector as well as the patient approaches of other disciplines like psychology, sociology, and anthropology are included in it. Therefore, there is no specific model to follow. However, every model should include patient and community at the core of each intervention.

The best cases are selected (case-based approach) including models, theories and strategies that can touch the hearts of the people, ensure their involvement in the ongoing probems, and chiefly, participate in working up solutions to facilitate the journey toward *better health*.

Piotrow, Rimon, Payne Merritt, and Saffitz identified four *"eras"* of health communication, shown below:

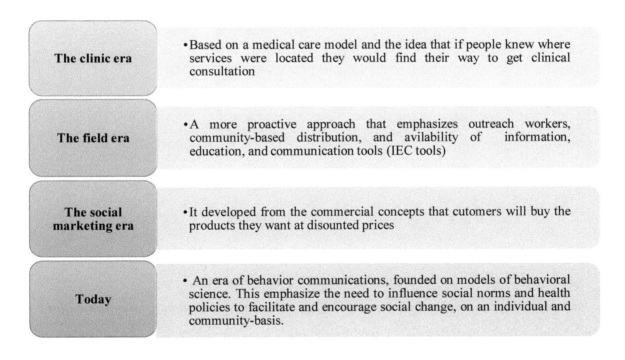

| The clinic era | • Based on a medical care model and the idea that if people knew where services were located they would find their way to get clinical consultation |

| The field era | • A more proactive approach that emphasizes outreach workers, community-based distribution, and avilability of information, education, and communication tools (IEC tools) |

| The social marketing era | • It developed from the commercial concepts that cutomers will buy the products they want at disounted prices |

| Today | • An era of behavior communications, founded on models of behavioral science. This emphasize the need to influence social norms and health policies to facilitate and encourage social change, on an individual and community-basis. |

Four eras of health communication

11

Many of the theoretical approaches of the different health communication eras still find a use in planning or execution of programs commercially e.g. situation analysis of a health communication program.

Certain stakeholders and opinion leaders may help communicators gather support by using the steps of *"McGuire's communication for persuasion"* (see figure below). It keeps the focus of the communicators focused on involving patients in the process and on the best possible health approach in influencing people's core beliefs. This practice enables the process to become really fluid and suited to cater to audiences' needs.

4. Strategic

Communication strategy can be defined as

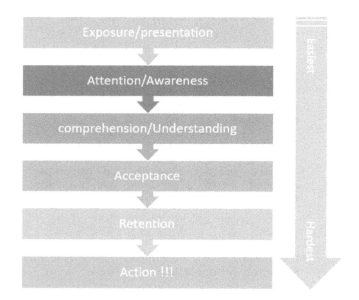

McGuire's Model of Persuasion (1984)

"the overall approach used for accomplishing objectives in healthcare communication"

Displaying effective strategies for health communication programs is really important and includes well-planned activities that respond to specific needs of the patients. Consider an example of Bethany, a 25-year old mother who is unsure about immunizing her newborn child. The communication between her and her health care provider is likely to affected in the following manner :

a. Bethany is likely to be influenced (at least, even significantly) by her health care provider and not by family or other new mothers

b. There may be some gaps in the patient' understanding that prevents health care providers from effectively communicating with the patient

c. Healthcare providers lack proper tools to talk about the concerned topic with patients in a timely and efficient manner.

Communication strategies need to be research based, where every activity is itself a strategy. Program planners should not rely heavily on specialized workshops, press releases, literature, flyers, or videos to provide effective communication. They should rather ensure that the content and format reflects the strategy) and prioritizes reaching the community's heart. Therefore, the strategies should respond to actual needs that have already been identifies by research and validated by the target population.

5. Process-oriented

As a long-term process, health communication Influences people and their attitudes through ongoing commitment to solving health issues. This originates from a deep understanding of patients in their environments and aim of building a consensus among members about the action plan. Evolution of such communication programs can occur due to the change in participant's input including patients, groups, professional organizations, policymakers, legislators, etc.

Process-oriented projects are often misunderstood in the midst of an ongoing health communication project despite of the fact that multiple channels and approaches are used. Such projects don't even rely solely on mass media. Process-oriented health communication strategies help the communicators in persuasion, involvement and development of consensus and feelings of ownership among the target population.

Let us look at an example. *"Exchange"* is U.K.-based networking and learning program on health communication for development and has multiple partners. It defines health communication as

"a process for partnership and participation that is based on two-way dialogue, where there is an interactive interchange of information, ideas, techniques, and knowledge between senders and receivers of information on an equal footing, leading to improved understanding, shared knowledge, greater consensus, and identification of possible effective action"

Communication for development relies on creative solutions to compensate for the lack of local capabilities and infrastructures and solutions emerge after months of discussion with local organizations, government officials and patient groups. Let us consider an example of Maria, a mother of four children who lives in a small village in sub-Saharan Africa with her 75-year old father. Her village is located remotely, isolated from major metropolitan cities and only a few literate people live there. Radios are also scarce. She is unaware that malaria (endemic in her area) is more dangerous for her children than elderly. As elders enjoy a better hierarchical position, even if Maria manages to buy mosquito nets (with difficulty), she will prefer that her father uses it and not her kids, leaving her children unprotected. Even though mortality rate among children due to malaria is quite high in her village, the village leaders advised her the opposite. If they had not, she would have likely chosen to protect her children. So her village leaders need to be involved to bring long-term changes in their community. It will require local involvement of organizations and authorities who also possess a respectable position in the eyes of community leaders. It also needs open minds to receive and act upon suggestions to find solutions to problems with the help of all stakeholders.

The lack of local capabilities ease of access to adequate communication channels, it will take much longer than similar projects in the developed countries. It is an ongoing process and even small steps should be appreciated.

6. Cost-Effective

The concept of "cost-effectiveness" in healthcare communication has been borrowed from commercial and social marketing. This is particularly important in nonprofit organizations where lack of funds and economic planning can affect initiatives, however, the problem can be dealt by using minimum human and economic resources. Communicators should make good use of their funds and advance their research-based strategy. Other creative solutions should also be sought to minimize the expenditure by seeking partnerships, using existing materials as starters, and increasing synergies with efforts of other departments in their organization or external groups.

7. Creativity in Support of Strategy

Creativity allows communicators to consider multiple options, methodologies, and channels to reach population by devising sustainable and cost-effective solutions for specific health communication interventions. However, even the best ideas can fail to attain psychosocial channels if they do not appeal to and endorsed by target population and key stakeholders.

Let us consider an example where brochures are provided to a community where malaria is endemic, about the use of insecticide-treated nets (ITNs). This activity seems logical only if the community is already aware of the malaria transmission cycle and the need for protection from mosquitoes. If they still believe in malaria being contracted by river-bathing or a complication of other fevers, the first step is *disease awareness* with focus on transmission cycle and preventive/protective measures. All activities should aim to share basic information before imparting specialized instructions like the use of ITNs and preferring them over other protection measures. It is the creative skill of the communicator to devise a culturally-suitable and appropriate tool engage community in behavior-modification attributable to the disease prevention. However, communicators should avoid developing and implementing sensational ideas that do not respond to actual needs of the community.

8. Audience and Media Specific

Audience and media specific health communication can be understood in the best possible way by revisiting the important lessons learned after the 2001 *"anthrax-by-mail" bioterrorism* that shocked the United States. The lethal agent *Bacillus anthracis* was mailed to senators and media personalities, packed in envelopes. Workers in the U.S. Postal Service facility in Washington were exposed to anthrax, out of which, two unfortunate workers died after inhaling anthrax spores

In that time of great emergency, the communication was found by several medical, patient, media and community representatives as well as public to be inconsistent and disorganized. Postal staff of U.S. Senate also reported their trust in public health agencies to be "eroded". The strategy was termed *"one message–one behavior approach"* caused postal workers in Washington to feel left out, majority of whom were African Americans or severely hearing impaired workers. That calls out for "relationship" or "rapport" development of public health officials with people belonging to different racial communities, underprivileged backgrounds, and those with physical limitations.

The learnt lessons from "anthrax scare" reinforce the support to the fundamental principles of effective healthcare communication. Information needs to be audience-specific and transmitted through effective channels. *One message–one behavior approach* should be avoided even with scarce time and resources.

9. <u>Relationship Building</u>

Communication is like a relationship: developing and nurturing good relationships is critical towards making health communication interventions successful. Such relationships must exist between all the stakeholders: patients, communities, health organizations, governments, and members of health teams. They can help build strong, long-term and successful coalitions, endorsement of stakeholders and increase in number of ambassadors to represent the health cause. Most importantly, "shared meanings and understanding" are created by good relationships that can bring psychological change at personal and community levels.

10. <u>Aimed at Behavioral and Social Change</u>

Today era is an era of "strategic behavior communications". Influencing behaviors and social norms through health communication is the ultimate goal but there is growing emphasis on establishing behavioral and social objectives at the earliest period of designing the health communication interventions.

Consider the different situations. Ask first: ***"What do you want people to do?"***, then: ***"do you want to get your children vaccinated before they turn two?"***, ***"are you aware of your risk for heart disease and would work to prevent it? Would they ask their dentists about oral cancer screening? Do they want stricter laws on the use of infant car seats? Or something about teenage smoking?*** Answers to these kinds of questions is the first step to establish research-based objectives of a communication program.

Social and behavioral change are two interconnected parameters: ***a series of behavioral changes precedes a social change.***

Health Communication in Public Health

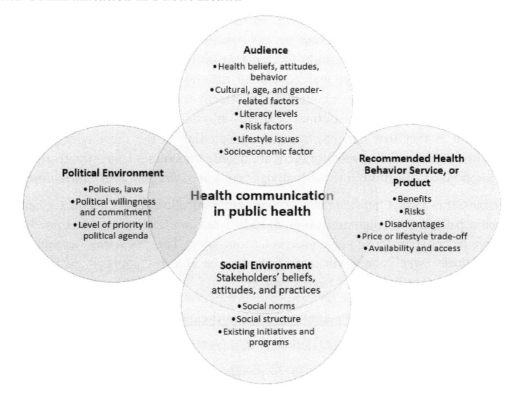

Health communication in public health

Despite the awareness at local and international levels, health communication has not been extensively used in public health, perhaps because it is considered as a skill rather than a distinct discipline. Fortunately, most public health organizations now recognize health communication as an important contributor to better health outcomes and general health status of populations in question. There is now awareness about interpersonal communications, professional medical communications, and public relations.

U.S. Department of Health and Human Services (2005), defines the U.S. public health agenda as

"health communication in public health includes disease prevention, health promotion, health care policy, and the business of health care as well as enhancement of the quality of life and health of individuals within the community. It holds a special place especially in the era of emerging infectious diseases, global threats, bioterrorism, and a new emphasis on a preventive and patient-centered approach to health"

Doctor-patient communication in multicultural settings:

Healthcare communication in *"multicultural settings"* is a field of particular interest for those involved. As the migration is increasing, access is required to important legal, medical and social services. There is a need of a multi-faceted approach involving health professionals and intermediaries. Extensive research has concluded that no matter how knowledgeable the clinician may be, if he or she cannot communicate effectively, then it is unlikely that they will be able to help that patient. Asnani defines "Patient – physician communication" as concludes that although it is fact that patient-physician consultation is the most widely performed 'procedure' in a clinician's life, most of them are unable to communicate effectively with the patient. Things take a disastrous turn when things take a *'multilingual and multicultural'* turn.

Language barrier is a great hurdle in one-on-one communication between a doctor/healthcare worker and a patient. This communication already lacks in effectiveness, imagine having a third person in between them – an interpreter/translator. The *"two-way"* communication changes to *"three ways"* communication. Can they be able to "connect" with each other without being able to talk directly? Seems unlikely.

Presentation in healthcare

Merriam-Webster Dictionary defines *"presentation"* as

"the act of presenting" or "the act, power, or privilege especially of a patron of applying to the ordinary for instituting someone into a benefice".

In other words, talking in professional terms, it is a "formal event" characterized by "teamwork" and "use of audio-visual aids". The basic purpose of presentation is *"sharing of information, persuasion of the audience for action and generation of goodwill".*

Presentation are one of the most important tools for effective communication in healthcare settings. The presentations are usually targeted at a larger audience e.g. the whole department, the whole administrative team, staff from all over the hospital, first year medical students of MBBS: this makes the **"presentations"** a very important way to share information with a large group of audience in a personalized way, and keep audience connected while expressing one's ideas.

To start, there are four fundamental requirements for any presentation to become a good presentation:

- A good subject matter
- Should match with the objective

- Should best fit the kind of audience
- Should be well organized

Presentations hold a very special importance in healthcare industry. In almost every aspect of healthcare, the art of presenting comes in handy.

The art of presentation - working with adult audiences

What is a person's first encounter with a presentation? School. Yes, everyone witnesses their first ever presentation when they are children. in schools, we got the chance to become audience of our teachers. And what and how we learned from our teachers, has certainly left a great impact on our lives, one way or another. As easy as it may sound, teaching anyone in general, is not easy, and teaching children in particular is a feat that deserves a lot of appreciation. From my view, the presenter is the "teacher" and the audience are the "students".

In healthcare presentations and other professional audiences however, our audience is not "children" but professional "adults". Working with adults is also difficult. We may have certain advantages on our side while working with adults: they can understand better, there are no comprehension issues, less problems with "age-appropriation" of content, etc.

To make children pay attention and concentrate on the academic presentation or lesson, a teacher can do certain things: action that involve both negative and positive reinforcement (reward and punishment, to be exact). In case of adults, the first, and the most important point that one has to understand, is that what worked with a child will not work with mature audiences. Therefore, strictly action-wise, time-outs, punishments and detentions cannot be used. But we can still use negative and positive reconditioning, in a different way. This is based on the concept of "adult learning".

Adult learning is *"distinct from child education, and is a practice in which adults engage in systematic and sustained self-educating activities in order to gain new forms of knowledge, skills, attitudes, or values"*

In adult learning, the teacher or presenter has to keep certain important things in mind. First, the structured information-sharing has to be done in a very limited time, say an hour (more than 40 hours of professional presentation are termed as excessive). Also, children are more vulnerable to change than adults. For presenting to adults, a more mature approach is needed.

One of the most important purposes of presenting on any occasion, particularly in healthcare setting is to practice **"persuasion"** and *"expression of ideas/opinions."*

The skill of persuasion in presentation – the importance of "powerful ideas":

Persuasion and *gaining influence* over the audience/ peers has never been more in demand than now, among healthcare workers and medical academics. Gone are the days when people could have been influenced by or expected to comply by simply asking them. Now the presented should be able to *"sell your ideas"*.

Having powerful ideas and be able to share or deliver them well are the keys to an effective and successful presentation. As money can buy you things, ideas can get you communication – *"ideas are the currency of communication"*.

In today's world of hustle and bustle and so many distractions, sharing information alone will never influence anyone to perform a certain task, or act in a certain kind of way. Only **"ideas"** have the power to persuade the people.

There is another word that had been used for *"power"* in the *old* times, and that is *"rhetoric"*.

Oxford dictionary describes "rhetoric" as

> *"the art of effective or persuasive speaking or writing, especially the exploitation of figures of speech and other compositional techniques"*

People have been taught the **"art of rhetoric"** since ancient times, to tell them how to assemble and deliver their ideas. Nowadays, at least in Europe, a few people study **"rhetoric"** systematically. However, the quality of persuasion can be drastically improved by the application of a few simple principles.

a) <u>Character, logic and passion</u>

The grandfather of rhetoric, Aristotle, claimed that we can persuade in two ways:

- Through the *"supporting evidence"* we can bring for our case
- And through *"artistic"* persuasion

Whatever we can bring for our case is the *"evidence"* – may include use of documents or witnesses; nowadays we may also bring research results or focus groups. **"Artistic"** persuasion possess three kinds of appeals which is the skill persuader himself uses:

Appealing to the audience's **reason**	Appealing to the audience's sense of your **character or reputation**	Appealing to the audience's emotions

Aristotle's named these three appeals as: *ethos, logos and pathos*. And they have become really well-known since then.

Logic (logos):

Logic always comes with rational thought - it is the work of conscious thinking. When we used "logos", we appeal to the audience's ability to reason. We do this by *constructing an argument*, *creating the reasons to support* the case we are making and *demonstrating how those reasons do so*.

There are two forms in which logic comes: *deductive* and *inductive*

Character (ethos)

It was quite early when rhetoricians realized that people could be swayed with the same intensity by *"passions and prejudices"* as by reason. For example, if we trust and respect someone, we will believe them and the things they say. Ethos is that appeal to our audience through reputation, personal credibility and the personality. *Why should the audience believe in what you are saying? What are your qualifications to comment on this matter? What is your expertise and how much experienced are you? How good is your reputation standing with them? How much value can you add to the argument from your experience?* The character of the persuader creates the trust upon which he or she can the argument.

Passion (pathos)

It is a fact that in the end, people are probably more influenced by their emotions than by anything else. Appealing to their feelings – pathos – is the most vital element in any attempt of persuasion. Unfortunately, attempt to appeal to emotions is sometimes mistaken for and condemned as *manipulation.*

The truth is, we cannot inspire emotions by just talking about it - we must present something external that will arouse them. An appeal for charity, e.g. might arouse or try to arouse people for donations by showing pictures of children dying in hospital, or animals in distress. Pathos has a reputation of being dishonest or unethical, however, this doesn't mean we should totally avoid it. Persuasion cannot be effective without emotion. The emotion need not be overwhelming, rather appropriate.

All three of these qualities: *character, reasoning and passion* must be present if you ever want to persuade people. The process of working out persuasion consists of five key elements:

1. Identification of the core idea

2. Logical arrangement of your ideas
3. Development of an appropriate style in the language
4. remembering the ideas
5. delivery of ideas with words, visual cues and body language (non-verbal behavior).

What's your message? What is your big idea?

If you want to persuade someone, first, you must have a message. Think about what do you want to say? A *single governing idea* is more likely to persuade your audience than a group of ideas, simply because one strong idea is easier to memorize. Focus. Begin by collecting thoughts and gathering ideas. Conduct imaginary conversations and note down the things who may end up saying. It is always better to jot down your ideas as they come and store them on a pad or in a file. Spend as much time as you can on this activity before the conversation itself. Then, ask these fundamental questions:

 i.   What is my main aim? What do I want to achieve? What would I call success?
 ii. What good I expect to happen?
iii. Who is going to be my audience? Why will be talking to them about this objective? What is their current knowledge about this topic? How much more do they need to know? What should they do? What kind of ideas will convince them? What is the most important thing I have to say to them?

People are only persuaded if the presenter's ideas interest them. The audience will only be interested in your ideas because they answer some query that exists in their minds.

A simple *four-point structure* will bring your audience to the point where accepting your message will be the only option left for them. Remember the letters **SPQR.**

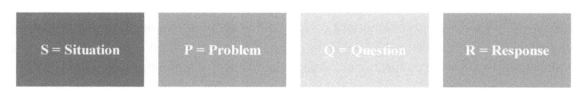

a) **Situation**

Start by briefly familiarizing the listener with things they already know – like a *"blast from the past"* – previous lecture topic, last week's journal club, your previous case presentation, etc. Make a statement that they will agree with – statement that relates to something that matters to them. This shows that you are *on their territory*: you understand their *situation*, circumstances and your appreciation of their point of view. Think of it as an opener *"Once upon a time…"* – a statement that describes what to expect next.

b) Problem

Now you should identify the problem that has come with the situation - the listener may or may not be informed/knowledgeable about the problem. However, it is customary for them to be aware of it. To be exact: *let the problem be their problem at least as much as yours*. There are many types of problems – many shapes and forms but it is vital to identify a problem that the listener will identify and must correspond with the situation. Some examples are:

- Something's gone wrong
- Something could change
- Someone has a different point of view
- We don't know what to do

Problems can be both positive and negative

c) Question

The Problem causes the listener to ask a *"question"*. If they do, be prepared to respond to them. If they don't, remind them that carefully that some questions are worth asking. *What do we do now? Which course should we take now? Etc.*

d) Response

Your *"response"* or reply to the question is basically your message. So, the message/idea should smoothly spring out as a logical and impactful answer to the question arising in the audience's mind by getting familiar with the problem.

SPQR is a classic framework which is a method frequently used by speakers and presenters. It is also helpful for important meetings, proposals and conversations. Taking the audience through the all four stages is the *"trick"* here.

Plan your presentation:

In planning your presentation, there are certain steps that need to be followed. Following these steps will give a better structure to the presentation and confidence to the presenter:

i. Define your objective

ii.   Identify your audience

iii.   Construct a message

iv.   Create a structure (**SPQR**, pyramid, etc.)

v.   Put it on cards

vi.   Add "spice"

vii.   Design visuals

viii.   Rehearse!!

Arrange your "ideas" – prepare your message:

Ideas are assembled and made coherent by logic. Every presenter must have a number of key ideas lined up that support the message.

Express your ideas:

Having the ideas coherently arranged in your mind is not enough to make an impact. A presenter has to bring the ideas alive in the audience's mind. It is better to use **"words"** that *"develop pictures and feelings"* to trigger their senses as well as thoughts.

Remember! We don't remember words during a presentation. We nearly forget what presenters say during a presentation but we tend to remember images. The images that retain in the memory are those which trigger the sensations and impressions. If you are successful in exciting your audience's imagination this way, your idea will be planted in their long-term memory.

Memory = (visuals) image + (emotions) feeling

You can create memories with your presentation through even only one of the five basic senses: *sight, hearing, touch, smell and taste.* To each his own: some people need to be convinced by pictures, some by powerful words while some want 'hands-on' demonstration.

Neuro-linguistic programming works on people's natural sensory preferences for receiving information. NLP develop this awareness of sensory preference into a systematic approach to communication via presentations!! Some examples are:

- Examples
- Stories
- Visuals
- Metaphors

Remember your ideas

Memory played a vital role in the art of presentation and persuasion. With no way to take notes and difficult to access books, in the past, remembering ideas was very critical in any presentation. That is why, whole systems of memory were created to help people store information and access it when they need it. *"Memory"* is not an important skill nowadays except during assessments and examinations - technology has replaced it. However, memory is still important when it comes to present something and convince people.

A successful presenter should find ways to bring the ideas off paper and into audience's head. Draw a colorful mindmap. Assemble a mental pyramid, scribble it and carry it. You can also use a notepad, a flip chart, a whiteboard. Invite the audience to join in, participate: encourage them to think.

Effective delivery of message:

"Delivery" signifies sharing your message with the support of effective behavior. If you will say one thing but your body is not agreeing with it, no one will believe your words. Think about the style of delivery audience may like. Is it up to audience if they like a relaxed and casual style of conversation or a more formal one? Delivery is about three kinds of activities. Concentrate on the way you use your: eyes, voice, body.

- **Maintain eye contact**

Eyes speak more than words. Maintaining eye contact with the audience is of vital importance. Try to include everybody with your eyes.

- **Use your voice**

The voice should not be too high, fast or thin. Learn to regulate and strengthen the breathing while you speak. Breathe deep and slow. Let your voice emerge more from your body than from your throat

- **Show a persuasive body language**

The face, the limbs and the body posture, all contribute to the total effect of your message on the listener. To start with, try to keep your face and neck muscles relaxed. Use your hands to paint pictures, to help you find the right words and express yourself fully.

Bibliography:

1. "Communicate." Merriam-Webster.com Dictionary, Merriam-Webster, https://www.merriam-webster.com/dictionary/communicate
2. "Health Communication: From Theory to Practice" by Renata Schiavo
3. Encarta Dictionary: English, North America.
4. "Improve your communication skills" by Alan Barker

CHAPTER 2

Tools for Health Communication

"The study and use of communication strategies to inform and influence individual and community decisions that enhance health."

Health Communication by "The Community Guide"

Overview:

There is no denying the importance of effective communication skills in healthcare. One critical step is identifying the tools which can be used for this purpose. We are living in the "Era of Technology". We have access to not just the print media and conventional media, but also the "social media".

In the health communication process, identifying the *"vectors" or "vehicles"* used for transmitting or relaying the information to the target audience, is the first and the foremost step. The tools must be chosen keeping in perspective the objectives that need to be met and the resources available to the health and administrative teams.

Nearly every person in the healthcare team thinks of himself as a good communicator, some think they are perfect. However, if a patients' survey is conducted and everybody gets to know about their communication skills coming uninterrupted from the patients, everyone would get to know, albeit discomforting, that we are far from perfect. Rather, we may be deficient in communication skills and lack in many aspects of our capability to 'give and take" information to and from the patients.

A research study evaluating the doctor-patient interaction concluded that most healthcare staff members will interrupt a patient every 16 seconds as he starts talking. Doesn't seem peculiar because there has to be a reason as to why less scores are always handed over to the doctors by the patients, especially when asked about their communications skills.

In the immediate future, it is expected that healthcare staff compensations will be given to them according to rating of their communications skills. An idea known as "Pay for

Performance" can be seen in lots of programs and they will base the compensations, at least partly, on patient satisfaction which is heavily dependent on provider's communication skills.

Basic tools of communication:

These tools are divided into 3 broad categories:

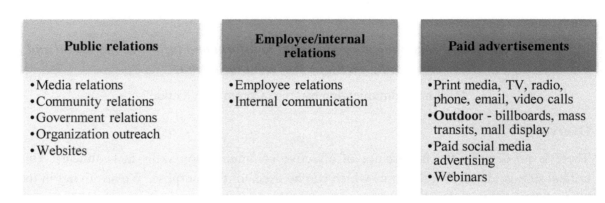

Basic tools in health communication

1. Public Relations:

The most important method of communication is a well-thought out and a steady, consistent plan of implementation for maintaining public relations. In addition, it is also the most cost-effective method of communication to this day. Over a long period of time, efforts for systematic public relations will make the survival of the organization possible, in every situation with an unaltered repute.

Let us look at the table below, showing tools required to establish and maintain the health communication with general public:

Public relation	Description of key components	Resources
Media relations	• Includes regular contact establishment with journalists (media alerts, feature articles, news releases, news conferences, seminars, background information kits, allocating a focal person/spokesperson, editorials and interviews).	• Time for the staff to develop and maintain a systematic media relations platform • Must follow organization's work plan • Direct and regular contact is a successful long-term approach

Community relations	• Consistent contact with individuals and organizations within the jurisdiction of the organization. • Includes speaking, other vocal engagements, presentations, civic and public group meetings, sponsorships, direct mails or newsletters.	• Staff time needed for coordination/arrangement of meetings and presentations. Time for attendance and follow-up. Some materials may be required for handouts or boards for display.
Government relations	• Direct, systematic and regular contact with public officials. • It may include personal contact, emailing, mailing, meetings, briefings	• Time for the staff to initiate relationships and maintain contact. For research or printing, some material may be needed.
Organization outreach	• It requires maintenance of organizational attendance at community events (special events, trade shows, community health fairs). • Includes displays, debates or presentations, focal person allocation to represent the organization.	• Time to organize events and assign representatives to attend for organization. Costs may be born for displays, brochures, handouts, giveaways
Websites	• Creation and maintenance of a web site to organize information regarding all programs and updated news. • It is an excellent source of information, education and an interaction for the stakeholders.	• Depends on organizational capabilities of the organization: may be design and engineering costs for initiation and maintenance. May work with internal IT support maintenance and development

Health communication tools for public relations

2. Internal/Employee relations:

A well-connected and a well-informed group of employees in terms of communication is an important contributor towards the success of any organization. In addition, the tools used for this communication need not be complex: most of them are very simple and low in cost, any are capable of enhancing public relations with assistance of the employees. The table below shows the description of such type of health communication tools:

Employee relations and internal communication	Description of key components	Resources
Employee relations	For employees, following guidelines should be followed: • Employees should be informed first • Employees should be provided with both written and electronic summaries of important, relevant information • Key contact person and suggested resources for more information should be provided • Allocate time to answer employees' questions as soon as possible	• Staff time • A commitment to ensure smooth flow of employee information
Internal communication	• Regular communication channels for the staff: may include emails, e-newsletters, staff meeting minutes, posters/digital posters, flyers, bulletin boards.	• Staff time • Minimum costs for printing costs • Developing the habit and accountability of content are important factors

Health communication tools for employee relations and internal communication

3. Paid advertisements:

Employee relations and internal communication	Description of key components	Resources
Print, radio, TV, phone, email, video messages	<ul><li>Paid advertisements in the media are certainly an effective strategy for any special event or even emergency situations</li><li>The size and frequency and advertisement placement should be planned carefully as it is important for optimal effectiveness</li><li>Generally, as far as advertisements are concerned, TV is the most expensive, radio is less expensive than TV and newspaper is the least expensive. Magazine or special publication ads may be effective if well targeted to your audience.</li></ul>	<ul><li>Costs are the highest for paid advertisement, however, they can be highly effective, as they have the ability to reach target audiences with relevant messages</li><li>Time is required to plan the time, place and distribution of advertisements, to appeal to the target audience.</li></ul>
Outdoor: billboards, mass transit, mall displays	<ul><li>Outdoor paid advertisement is always planned as a part of a comprehensive campaign: this is a really effective advertising strategy.</li><li>It is important to align the advertisements to the needs and interest of the audience, and make sure that the advertising money is being used in the best way</li></ul>	
Paid advertisements on social media	<ul><li>Social media applications like facebook, Instagram, twitter, whatsapp, youtube and many others are also used to promote and propagate ideas related to health education.</li><li>Many health facilities, individual teams and clinicians employ the marketing companies who offer paid subscriptions to them, to promote their message on the social media.</li></ul>	
Webinars	<ul><li>Webinars are adopted as a tool of communication, comparatively recently, since the advent of COVID-19 pandemic.</li><li>Nowadays, many health seminars, training sessions, discussions, even international conferences are conducted online via webinars</li></ul>	

Health communication tools for employee relationships and internal communication

Summary:

Research-based strategies are used to advertize materials and health products; select the pathways that can be used to deliver them to the target audience.

Conventional insights, concepts, priorities and languages are understood and employed to appeal to multicultures communities and neighborhoods.

The health literacy, access of people to internet facitilties, media coverage and cultural competency of intended cohorts is taken into consideration

This also includes searching for relevant medical literature and preparation of materials for propagation e.g. brochures,newspaper articles, pamphlets, billboards, TV broadcasts, radio commercials, public service messages, newsletters,, videos, other digital tools, case studies, health fairs, and field trips among others.

A variety of communication methodologies are used that allow messages pertaining to health to tailor media, personal, small group, large group or community level campaigns. the purpose of such strategies is to change people's perception, knowledge, attitudes, and behavior

- Attempts to increase risk perception of the population
- Positive reinforcement of agreeable behaviors
- Bringing positive changes to social norms
- Easy and immediate availabiliy of support and beneficial services
- Encourage and promote healthy behaviors to improve health conditions
- Some examples of successful media strategies to transmit health messages are:
  - Radio, TV, organizational newsletters, newspapers, health posters, flyers, brochures, internet. social media tools (Twitter, Facebook, YouTube, etc.)

Some examples of **successful interventions** in health communication:

- Programs for tobacco prevention and cessation which are often targetted to reach a wider audience (mass-reach) - e.g. *"Rural Tobacco Control and Prevention Toolkit"* initiative in the U.S.
- HIV prevetion and treatment strategy was implemented through social media marketing interventions available as *"Rural HIV/AIDS Prevention and Treatment Toolkit"* in the U.S.

Communication in health includes employment of verbal and written strategies to influence and authorize individuals, neighborhoods, populations, communities and nations to make wholesome and healthier choices. Health communication blends multiple, individual theoretical components of health models to boost favorable changes in attitudes and behaviors of masses. Health communication is related to social marketing, which involves the development of activities and interventions designed to positively change behaviors. Social marketing methodologies helpful in effective communication in healthcare are mentioned in the image.

Awareness can also be brought to the population through screening by organization of free health camps. In the U.S. state of Louisiana, ***The Northeast Louisiana Regional Pre-Diabetes Prevention Project*** promoted prediabetes screening and prevention information to communities in the vicinity by using multiple media outlets.

We have recently experienced COVID-19 pandemic in the 21st century. The role of media, whether print, electronic or social media, played pivotal roles in educating the masses about the prevention and treatment of the disease. Same effective communication strategies have helped curtail the problem by achieving "herd immunity" by mass vaccinations, which would not have been possible without the assistance of media campaigns and promotions. Both state-dependent and independent media outlets, all over the world, participated in it.

Considerations for utilization of health communication tools

When designing health communication or social marketing strategies, it is important to consider the overall communication goals of the intervention. It is also necessary to understand the target population so that the content created is relevant to the target population. It is important to tailor messages to the communication channel being used. Further, using multiple communication and media strategies will ensure a broader reach. It is also important to ensure that the target population has access to the communication channels being used.

<u>An example of using inexpensive and accessible communication tools to help provide health education to underprivileged parts of the world</u>

A research study conducted as a part of an investment plan by *"**Bill and Melinda Gates Foundation**"* for supporting the government of Indian state of Bihar, to help them improve ***Reproductive, Maternal, Newborn and Child Health and Nutrition (RMNCHN)*** throughout the state. ***BBC Media Action*** was trusted to implement the communication tools. These tools supported ***front-line worker's outreach***. They analyzed the effect of a package of *"mHealth audio messaging"* and *"paper-based job aids"* used by front line workers during the sponsored ***village health, sanitation and nutrition days (VHSNDs)*** on KAPs (knowledge, attitude and practices) of women of childbearing age within the RMNCHN program limitation.

This study titled ***"Implementing health communication tools at scale: mobile audio messaging and paper-based job aids for front-line workers providing community health education to mothers in Bihar, India"*** was published in British Medical Journal. It concluded that:

"As technology advances and smart phones become more ubiquitous, even in hard-to-reach places, a rich opportunity has emerged for the delivery of quality healthcare through mHealth interventions. Our analysis has shown that implementation of digital and non-digitally facilitated communication tools for FLW support are associated with higher levels of self-reported knowledge and healthy behaviors, as well as subsequent discussions with others in the family. Further study is required, however, to understand how mHealth tools can be utilized most effectively, and in what contexts. For instance, assessments should address whether digital health tools are more effective than paper-based visualization tools, particularly for supporting less educated or marginalized groups; or when and for what topics digitally facilitated communication is superior to direct-to-beneficiary digital tools. Only then can digital and mHealth assessments be optimized in their evidence-based use for purpose. Importantly, future evaluations of the effectiveness of mHealth interventions must also focus on health outcomes, and the long-term sustainability of health-related improvements. Technology tools continue to create opportunity for improved health impacts at scale, but their use must be evidence-based to ensure cost-effective implementation and sustained benefits for their beneficiaries"

Training Tools for effective communication for doctors

Training tools, or the tools which train doctors in communicating effectively, have been deeply embedded in medical education over the course of history. They have traditionally been taught with "practical skills" for teaching, where they have assisted in demonstrations related to anatomy and familiarizing medical students with technique of performing procedures. Various approaches exist, ranging from demonstrating on human cadavers, animal models, and specimens, to using simulations and simplified tools.

The training tools in the field of health communication have many proven benefits. They encourage and promote clear, uninterrupted communication and preclude the dire consequences that may arise from poor communication. After development, these training tools have been in use in multiple sectors and organizations (e.g. aviation industry) leaving a strongly positive impact in every sector. The positive reports coming in from non-medical sectors have helped provide much needed insight into the professional requirements of individuals and groups working in other challenging sectors. So, some of these tools, after being developed in other sectors, have ultimately found their way after they were analyzed and tailored for use in medical education. Therefore, the use of such tools in medical education and health sector is now a reality, which help curtail communication errors and improve delivery of healthcare.

Assessment of Procedural Skills

Simulation training has played an important role in medical education. It is self-explanatory as to why these training tools have to become an integral part of medical education. A medical student must learn to communicate effectively while he is still in the medical school, so that he may not put himself and others in any difficult situation due to lack of communication skills. Same holds true for house officers, postgraduate trainees, junior and senior registrars.

According to one review article in medical education, training in medical simulation produced positive effects on a trainee's learning, knowledge, and procedural skills. Additionally, it was of the view that these positive effects will likely be transferred into clinical practice. Additionally, not only that individual but the whole team gets benefitted from the simulation training as it promotes team compatibility and reduces the chances of error. It improves positive patient

Multiple training tools now exist for use, particularly within the simulation to improve both team and individual communication skills. Based on research, some communication tools for doctors are:

a) <u>Appropriate assertion tool:</u>

This tool specifically deals with "assertion" or involving "confidence" within cross-professional interaction. It is usually a nurse's responsibility to contact the doctor for requesting a patient visit. However, sometimes, this communication between doctors and nurses becomes difficult. Therefore, to address this lapse in communication, a cyclical process was developed with various stages:

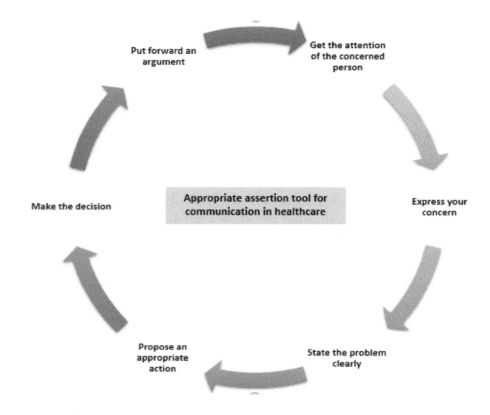

Put forward an argument → Get the attention of the concerned person → Express your concern → State the problem clearly → Propose an appropriate action → Make the decision

Appropriate assertion tool for communication in healthcare

Appropriate assertion tool for healthcare communication

b) Huddles

Implementation of huddles is another important tool which can be defined as "a tool which is used for communicating any changes in a plan of care." They are a multidisciplinary tools set at specific intervals that allows the group to focus within a staff shift or after any event. Usually, they require a general structure:

Huddle in an emergency department: a brief huddle (< 5 minutes) every hour to review patients with minor ailments, check if the plans are still in place and "alarm" is raised if any safety issue/deterioration comes up about a patient.

Set times, for example start and end of shift or an hour during shift	Mandatory attendance (all staff)	For a limited time (usually <15 mins)	Structural clarity and uniformity (every huddle should follow the same structure)

c) Debriefing:

Debriefing can involve both teams and individual members. It is another tool which aims at making the communication better, especially during the simulation methods. Its usually a a two-way discussion between facilitator and student at the end of a simulation session.

Effective communication tools for nurses:

In nursing care, effective communication is undoubtedly "the" most important skill where medical information need to be shared in detail, by the nurses with the patients, their primary caregivers, other staff members and clinicians. This communication has to be done, often at greatly stressful times. To ensure good quality personalized care to the patients through nursing care, good communication is critical. The ability to establish effective communication strategies and good attitude of the medical staff are by far the two most important factors contributing to high levels of patient care and satisfaction. However, there can be serious repercussions of having "breakdowns" in nursing communication.

Most nurses usually do have a good basic level of communication and nursing skills, but no harm comes to those who want to improve. By hard work and smart use of nursing communication tools, not only they can improve their job satisfaction, boost their morale and ensure patient care.

Methodologies and communication Tools for Nurses

Some smart strategies have been developed for the nurses to communication effectively with their patients and achieve better patient engagement, interactions, information sharing and smooth communication with other staff members. Through the use of these methods, nurses can become better communicators and the chances of medical errors and negligence will reduce.

SBAR Nursing Communication Tool		
Communication tool	Description and details	Examples
"SBAR" Acronym of:	• One of the commonest tools used in nursing for initiating and maintaining conversations. • It is used to ensure structured communication	**Situation:** state the name, ward, location, patient name and brief description of information, e.g. *"I am Martha in Cardiology ward on 4th floor calling about Mr. Collins, because his pressures are dropping"*.

S = Situation B = Background A = Assessment R = Recommendation	for information transfer to accurately occur between two people e.g. during a nursing shift change • It uses quick questions in 4 areas to help start and guide the conversation. Also to ensure accurate and effectual transfer of relevant information, e.g.:	**Background**: brief details of the background problem are provided, e.g. *"Mr. Collins was admitted yesterday with acute anterior wall STEMI"*
		Assessment: Provide brief account of your assessment, e.g. *"I have assessed this patient and I am worried about him because he looks really sick, I am not sure of the problem but he seems to be deteriorating"*
		Recommendation: give recommendations, e.g. *"I need to ask you to reach and see the patient in the next 10 minutes. Please let me know if I can do anything in the meantime before you reach?"* **NOTE:** The nurse initiating the conversation should ask the responder to repeat the important information in order to check if it has been understood

"BATHE" Protocol for Nursing

Communication tool		Description and details	Examples
BATHE protocol Acronym for: **B = Background** **A = Affect** **T = Troubles** **H = Handling** **E = Empathetic** **Statement**	• Much like SBAR, ***BATHE protocol*** serves as a prompt for four questions • Interaction is usually 1-2 minutes long (maximum 5 minutes) • Purpose: it is not meant for problem-solving or conflict resolution or to provide treatment. It is to give reassurance to the patient, deescalate the stress situation, and strengthen the nurse-patient relationship • This strategy has been trialed in an OPD setting with promising results so far: improvement in patient experience has been reported.	**Background**: *"What is going on in your life? How are things"* **Affect**: *"How is rheumatoid arthritis affected your life?"* **Troubles**: *"What is causing trouble in this situation, is getting out of bed too difficult now?"* **Handling**: *"How are you coping with it?"* **Empathetic Statement**: *"That must be really difficult for you and very frustrating too"*	

Communication tools in nursing based on technology

a) Mobile devices

Mobile devices are commonly used as they have been embraced by the people in healthcare industry due to quick and easy access. They are reliable and can help to open effective communication channels with patients. In the U.S., in some hospitals like the University of San Francisco Medical Center, they have purchased *tablets* to use at bedsides of the patients which provide information about the healthcare team members to the patients and also provide health education. Staff can designate relevant videos to the patients for watching to help in their recovery from health conditions. The devices can also send information to nursing offices and explain why they need staff attention without having to rely on call lights.

b) Institutionally-compliant SMS platform

Out of all the technical communication tools in modern times, text messaging platform is the most advantageous. Analogous to Whatsapp, this consumer instant messaging platform could incorporate a wide spectrum of features to improve communication between healthcare team and the patients.

This platform must only be used to send concise, essential information about patients e.g. results of investigations, relevant medical images, and details of patient conversations. Such tools can instantly contact specific individual team member and arrange its consultation. Correct information will be passed on to other staff during shift changes. Nurses can also check up on patients after a stay in the hospital stay. There is one-on-one correspondence and interaction via text, voice, or video call in group chats. The institutes that have already implemented this as a tool for communication tool are of the view that significant improvements have occurred in overall efficiency of the health system, staff productivity, patient understanding and satisfaction. Overall, duration of hospital stays has decreased, patient input has increased, chances of medical errors have lessened, and patient outcomes have improved.

Ticket-to-ride	• It is the most widely used tool for communication for patient handovers/transfer in nursing care • e.g. when a patient is transfered to radiology department for getting an X-ray, the patient is handed over to the transporter by the nurse and the information is provided • In other scenarios e.g. if the patient requires an IV or a wheelchair. This shows that the person in charge of the patient's care even for a brief period of time, is careful and possesses all the relevant information to keep patient safe.
Hourly rounds	• It involves arranging and conducting hourly visits to each patient's room or bedside • It is done to check up o their status or to ask if they need anything. different members of the team can conduct these • The task may seem difficult but its not if one is proactive and addresses the patient's needs before any emergency situation arises. it can save valuable time and makes patient care easy • It boosts patient satisfaction and improves overall experience.
Patient Teach-Back	• It is a good communication methodology to ensure patient understanding of the information imparted by a nurse. the nurse shares and expains a set of instructions/imformation and requests the patient to explain it all back • This helps the patient to register the information. Nurses should explain that this is not a test, but a communication tool that will help nurses assess patients' clarity of undestanding.
A Self-Check Checklist	• An aspect not to be overlooked is the nurses' own mental and physical state which can affect their ability to make rght decisions, have effective communicate and steer clear of errors • **TeamSTEPPS** devised a checklist called **"I'M SAFE" - Illness, Medication, Stress, Alcohol/drugs, Fatigue, Eating and Elimination** • If any of the items are not checked in e.g. *E – not eaten or A - too much alcohol*: that information is communicated to colleagues, as potential for errors increases in such situations

Some other tools for nursing communication are:

Sources:

1. University of North Dakota (ruralhealth.und.edu/communication/tools)
2. ruralhealthinfo.org/toolkits/health-promotion/2/strategies/health-communication
3. Ward V, et al. BMJ Global Health 2021;6:e005538. doi:10.1136/bmjgh-2021-005538
4. Rayner HM, Wadhwa R. Communication Training Tools in Medical Simulation. [Updated 2022 Jul 25]. In: StatPearls [Internet]. Treasure Island (FL): StatPearls Publishing; 2022 Jan-. Available from: https://www.ncbi.nlm.nih.gov/books/NBK560868/
5. hipaajournal.com/communication-tools-in-nursing/

CHAPTER 3

Why Communication in Healthcare is Important?

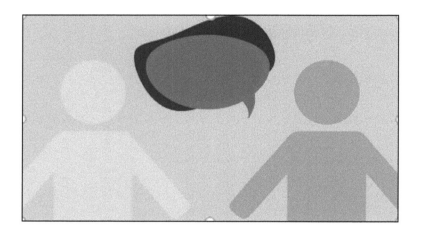

"Today's healthcare environment makes good communication among patients, families, and caregivers harder and harder to achieve. Hospital stays are shorter, medical care is more technologically complex, resources are constrained, and there is a growing need for patients and families to have more information about, and involvement in, care decisions."

American Hospital Association

Acute or chronic disease and injuries can affect life of any person dramatically and disrupt it to various extents. A patient expresses a whirlwind of emotions while fighting an illness or injury, as a reaction. This can lead to instability, impassivity and a feeling of dreariness.

For example, someone is being diagnosed with cancer which can take a person through a plethora of emotions in a single moment. There is the "fear" of the "unknown", feeling of having lost all control, perplexity, anger, grief, depression and anxiety can strike. Now the question arises: who will be there to help this person during this melancholic and perturbing time?

One's communication skills, as a healthcare professional are required to be stellar and a top priority. "All" healthcare professionals need good communication skills. The skill is not to be learnt by just the psychologists and social workers.

Some examples of good communication skills are: active listening, appropriately responding to patient's concerns and requirements, proper assessment of body language and carrying a non-judgmental attitude: which are all important skills that every healthcare worker must harbor inside of them. Giving the healthcare communication the importance it deserves in the domain of patient care, countless injuries and deaths can be prevented. Moreover, it multiplies the magnitude of trust between the patient and the healthcare provider. It also fortifies the patient's relationship with other members of the healthcare team, responsible for providing effective care to them. Not only can optimum health communication save lives in healthcare, it can also raise the chances of the staff amassing higher success rates on the job. Therefore, this is a two-way road.

It has been learnt from various research studies and feedback observation continuously over decades that a doctor's ability to listen, communicate and understand makes the recovery of the patients, swift and effective. Apart from recovery, an empathetic doctor affects the overall healthcare experience and satisfaction of the patient. However, that is not supposed to make other healthcare staff "relieved" from the responsibility. Caring for a patient in a hospital is mostly a multidisciplinary approach which almost always involves doctors and nursing staff. Not only the healthcare staff is responsible for maintaining fluent communication with the patients and caregivers, but also amongst each other.

Effective healthcare communication with the patients give them a feeling of empowerment and allows their family members to eagerly participate in their care as responsible partners. This can lead to improvement of treatment compliance and self-management.

Such supportive evidence sprouting from decades of research and observations fortifies the correlation between healthcare communication and desired healthcare goals. Thus, a "structured" channel of communication can markedly improve delivery of healthcare.

Reaching out to a hospital or clinic while suffering from any disease, the patients usually go through a lot of emotions. In healthcare setups, the situations are always far from perfect. not facing any problem, minor or major, is inevitable. Be it patient's entry, first contact with healthcare personnel, history taking, clinical examination, diagnosis, prescription writing and reassurance, disappointments are bound to happen. Every healthcare worker must know about the problems patients could experience. A lot of patients are going through anger and frustration at how the things may have come out for them. Some patients receive their "bad news" or "poor prognosis" news while they are still in the healthcare setups. That is where empathy is important. Communication is the key to show that empathetic response to the patients.

The importance of health communication does not limit itself to the hospitals but extends far beyond any healthcare setup. When the patients have leave the inpatient setting and shift out from under the care of healthcare staff, it is the duty of their designated healthcare team to continue to support them by keeping in touch with the patients. The communication must continue to ensure that the health outcomes are being met and their safety is not compromised. It is desirable for the care teams to maintain a strong, meaningful relationships with the patients and their care providers.

Current Issues in Health Care – Why Health Communication is important?

There are a lot of issues involving health care: a lot of them are specific to a certain country, environment, political situation, health issue or population, among others. Here are some examples of some current issues that are currently influencing health communication practice.

1. <u>Health Disparities:</u>

Health equity is a primary guiding principle for health organizations and signifies the importance of eliminating health disparities by removing differences in the well-being and health status of diverse populations. As Dr. Martin Luther King Jr. has said,

> *"Of all forms of inequality, injustice in health is the most shocking and the most inhuman"*

The US National Institute of Health define health disparities as the *'differences in the incidence, prevalence, mortality, and burden of diseases and other adverse health conditions that exist among specific population groups in the United States'"*

In practice, they refer to quality of health care as well as overall access to health services and products among different populations or subgroups of the same population, resulting in unfavorable patient outcomes or reduced life expectancy. some of the factors contributing to health disparities are listed in the figure.

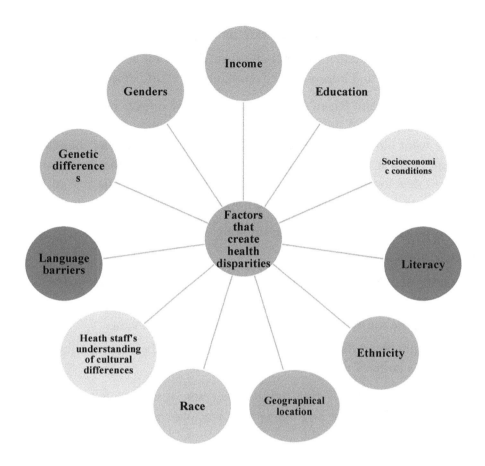

Factors that create health disparities

Audience-specific campaigns and programs and cultural competence (to relate to the unique characteristics of each population/ethnic group and to address) are requirements to eliminate health disparities.

2. Patient Empowerment

It refers to *"patient awareness about his disease and available treatment options which allows patients to hold informed discussions with doctors and participate in treatment/prevention decisions".* Patient empowerment can result in better patient compliance to treatment/prevention measures or development of healthy behaviors leading to improved health outcomes by getting involved in policymaking, healthcare legislations, medical practices, research funding, and social change.

3. Limits of Preventive Medicine and Habits

Unfortunately, preventive medicine cannot eliminate disease but it can contribute significantly to extend life expectancy and improve the overall quality of life of many populations.

Take an example of a Puerto Rican man who is a habitual smoker who is being pressured to quit by his family because of the oral cancer scare and wanting him to have regular doctor checkups. They want him to see doctor for prevention of cancer rather than in some serious illness. A recent death in the close family alarmed the family as the deceased was a heavy smoker who had developed oral cancer. However, Eduardo says that one of his very good friends developed oral cancer despite being a nonsmoker. He presented several arguments:

- There is no guarantee that quitting smoking will prevent oral cancer
- He enjoys smoking and drinking
- His family should not be worried about oral cancer as what happened to their deceased relative was very rare
- He has no time for busy for regular checkups with his doctor

Eduardo may be right about the limitations of preventive medicine, but, a few facts may help him see his family's point of view:

- Oral cancer incidence is two times higher among Puerto Rican men than among mainland U.S. Hispanics and higher than that observed in white males living on the mainland United States
- Tobacco together with alcohol is a primary risk factor for oral cancer (additive effect).
- Smoking cessation is a known preventive measure against oral cancer risk

It is important to keep in mind the unawareness of most people regarding risk factors, statistics and prevention of a disease. Prevention does not always work but it works in most of the cases.

4. The Emergence of E-Health

Internet and related technologies have expanded the "scope" of health care beyond conventional boundaries and has affected health communication, significantly. Patient, primary carers, healthcare staff, etc., all rely on internet for advice on health issues, pharmacies, health information systems and health records. Increased reliance on internet opened the way towards interactive health communication tools (Web sites, games, press rooms, disease simulations, opinion polls, seminars, etc). It has raised questions about the legitimacy of information on the Internet, its implications of patient privacy and equal information access by those who may not have the resources or skills to take advantage of new resources.

5. Low Health Literacy

It is the inability to read, understand and act on health information. It is one of the most important problems in health communication. The information, no matter how accurate, compelling, or appealing, the overall purpose seems to be defeated if people cannot understand it. It affects all different age groups and ethnic backgrounds. About 90 million Americans and significant population of Canada lacks basic literacy skills to understand health information. Low health literacy may include inability to write, read or solve basic math, and

- Poor speaking, listening, or comprehension capability
- Language barriers
- Low self-advocacy for oneself
- Inability to navigate the health care system
- Inadequate background information
- Low socioeconomic status

More recently, internet as an accessible source of information has divided those who take benefit from this situation, and those who don't. healthcare communication interventions can help sensitize health care workers, public health officers, institutional health representatives, and others about the need to reach out to patients and public in their own terms.

6. Impact of Managed Care and Other Cost-Cutting Interventions on Health

"Managed care" and "cost-cutting" interventions are being implemented in a lot of places around the world, especially in Asia where organizations manage the costs and healthcare delivery to patients. Many aspects of health care are now scrutinized/influenced by managed care. Both the health providers and patients should put forward their opinions on cost-saving interventions and their likely impacts. Health communication can help establish an environment where everyone will feel forced to *balance quality of care and cost-saving*, through advocacy, mass media campaigns, professional and government relations.

7. Reemergence of Communicable Diseases

Many diseases which had disappeared have reemerged and that has influenced health communication in two related ways:

It has led to *renaissance of health communication*: rising reemerging diseases cholera and tuberculosis, this communication should help raise awareness of the ongoing health risk. In fact, many infectious diseases may become a threat to the public again. Reemergence of *polio* or *Haemophilus influenzae type B* (meningitis and acquired mental retardation). Parents have been refusing childhood vaccinations. Five cases of polio reemerged in an Amish farm in Minnesota in 2005. These are strong reminders that vaccine-preventable diseases are also a threat worldwide, even the developed world. Communicating about the risks for infectious diseases is strategically very important.

8. The Threat of Bioterrorism

This kind of health threat has compelled all the stakeholders involved in the process of health communication to review and revise their strategies in the light of bioterrorism risk, e.g. lessons learnt from averting a potential public health disaster from the 2001 anthrax-by-mail attacks in the US. This includes:

- Message for the target audience should be claear, timely, specific and accurate
- Health representatives should be credible
- Planning should be strategic, efforts should be coordinated in the presence of adequate communication channels with culturally competent attitude

In emergencies, the issue of preparedness in really important.

9. Capacity and Infrastructure Building in the Developing World

Health communication cannot magically replace the lack or absence of local infrastructure, capacity, or training. However, health communication interventions can create sociopolitical willingness to build hospitals, strive to find resources, recruit and train local health workers. Nevertheless, it remains a major issue in developing countries.

Direct & effective communication and its importance for the healthcare team

A good healthcare team always operates by the utilization of open and reliable communication channels. Good communication is of prime importance when discussing clinical procedures, patient's requirements, and all the relevant information pertaining to the patients: clinical histories and detailed account of previous illnesses, treatments, etc. When important information is let to slip and fall through the cracks, there is a high chance that significant morbidity, mortality and malpractice will be avoidable.

Some healthcare institutes in the US have created certain information sharing and exchanging platforms that aim at making the patient care better through the use of organized systems. May examples can be given to explain how effective this can be, but, let's start with information exchange between two shifts of nurses during shift changes. The process can surely be long and dismaying. Due to this lengthy exchange of information about every patient between themselves, first contact of the new nurse with the patients is delayed by hours. Also, often during shift changes of doctors and nurses, patients feel as if they are being "ignored" and not looked after well, as the new staff will take time to reach them. If a problem arises during that time, patients feel that they are left "alone" to deal with them. To make the matters even more abysmal, the information exchanging process is neither always organized, nor systematic. Sometimes, healthcare staff are too busy to jot down each and every detail about all the patients. So some vital information can be missed from being shared. Many patients end up being provided things unnecessarily that they have already been provided while some patients are left to wonder why nobody came to check up on them. Imagine a patient whose vital signs got monitored twice and another one did not get checked even once. So, an organized system and a proper procedure for exchanging high-priority information swiftly and reliably, was developed: **Nurse/Doctor Information Exchange**. This different communication process makes sure that the information exchange happens in patient's rooms/wards at their bedsides, rather than on the nurses' counter. This will certainly take the patients into the fold and give them a feeling of being "involved" in the whole process. This will also reiterate the same principal of not letting any valuable patient information slip through the cracks and will potentiate the patient's trust on the system.

There are many different types of software that facilitate good communication and allows staff to go through notes; review, discuss and share information. Communication should be direct when the staff is dealing with accounting, billing and supervisors. Staff has to ensure that all the relevant healthcare staff (juniors and seniors, both) are a part of the whole process and not kept aloof.

There are many ways in which establishment of an effective communication with patients is important for healthcare workers.

Working with patients and their primary caregivers

It is essential that every healthcare worker reminds himself from time to time and keeping his work persona aside that he is working with human being, people who may be going through dilemmas of their own. Being unwell and being dependent on healthcare staff for diagnosis and treatment is a big challenge. A doctor should always commence the sessions with rapport-building and gaining trust of the patient. Words and expressions showing compassion, empathy and a non-judgmental attitude can help determine the true requirements of the patients as well as minimize or abolish mistrust, unnecessary issues. Same approach should be initiated with the immediate family members.

Providing the patients some simple education is essential. A doctor should be prepared to leave out fancy medical jargon until very necessary and explain the meanings of difficult words. Details regarding any medical or surgical procedures that may be difficult to understand, should be shared. All this should be carried out without getting annoyed and expressing frustration at the questions raised by patients or their family members. A doctor is always advised to conduct discussions at a reasonable pace, not very hurriedly and have patience. One should always imagine one's own self instead of the patient and try to step into the patient's shoes to increase empathy. Contrastingly, a doctor is never to keep the patients or their caregivers "in the dark" because this can cause a great deal of stress when things will come out into the light for them. Their anger will justifiably be skyrocketed.

Best Practices to Implement in healthcare communication:

a) <u>Understanding needs of different patients as different personalities:</u>

Every human being Is unique and so are the patients. During their careers, doctors come in contact with patients having different personalities or a "wide spectrum of personalities" ranging from pleasant to somewhat "difficult". Generally, the pleasant ones are the most effortless to communicate with. However, dealing with "difficult" personalities can be an uphill task, demanding patience. Remember this rule of thumb: always make sure one doesn't respond or react harshly or aggressively, because they are still patients who need understanding, and care. They deserve empathy even when they don't act like they deserve it and are not demonstrating any positivity in their responses despite your attempts. Kindness can really pave the way forward for them: their silver lining.

b) <u>Showing empathy</u>

According to Cambridge English dictionary, empathy can be defined as *"the ability to share someone else's feelings or experiences by imagining what it would be like to be in that person's situation"*. Empathy requires honesty and sincerity. It needs a deep connection to be established with the patients. Facial expressions are also essential to show empathetic feelings of kindness, patience, concern and calming effect. If a doctor or a nurse expresses "unreal" emotions and "fake" gestures, the patients will definitely notice. They will understand that the staff is not really concerned about them and are not extending true, genuine care. Empathy is walking through the patient's shoes as if you are the patient yourself. like a person seldom judges oneself, a doctor should not judge the patients and must dig deeper into their problems.

c) <u>Using active listening skills</u>

The United States Institute of Peace defines active listening as a way of listening and responding to another person that promotes mutual understanding. It is a vital first step to handle certain difficult situations and attempt problem solving. It is only through active listening that we can succeed in handling disagreements.

Using the mind and heart, not just the ears are required for active listening. Only via listening actively, one can recognize and understand a patient's hints, needs, phrases and expressions which mostly indicate discomfort, agitation, depression and other strong emotions. The key is to "listen more and talk less". Open-ended questions, free f interruptions should be asked from the patients, keeping in mind that the patients are observing your body language. Trick is to not appear defensive or nonchalant.

d) <u>Practicing note-taking</u>

Being ignorant about important patient information because it was not written down can really be unfortunate and one of the worst things that can happen: disastrous for the health facility. It is always advisable to take neat, relevant and concise notes. Same applies to notes being uploaded on a computer: one communicates with everyone involved in the patient care directly or indirectly via reading the notes. So note-taking is a communication tool which can be used to keep the members of the healthcare team to keep each other updated about the individual patient situations. Notes can include details regarding medication, signs and symptoms, past or recent medical or surgical procedures, specialized dietary and psychosocial needs are of prime importance in healthcare. Never become overconfident about it and put blind faith into your memory even if you think it is really eidetic.

e) <u>Always being direct and straight-forward</u>

Always be open and candid about everything that revolves around the patients, their families and caregivers. Never let any important information fall through the cracks in the system. There is never any room for errors and second chances do not exist – guesses don't work either. Communication models should be focused and transparent.

Direct communication in healthcare is the key to successful for carrying out routine operations irrespective of the role of a particular person in the team, it is a team effort. In a healthcare team, it is everyone's responsibility to keep communication channels up and running as good communication can actually save lives.

Having a good understanding of patients' needs and condition:

As a doctor, one should have a clear understanding of the patient's condition. For this, one should establish an effective communication with the patients – "establishing rapport". This focuses on how effectively the one-to-one correspondence happens between the doctor and the patients or their caregivers.

Sometimes, to ease the patient out and "break the ice", some doctors may need to ask personal details from a patient: about professions, family, hobbies, etc. After the patient becomes comfortable and rapport has been established, relevant and detailed history is asked. History taking is an important aspect of communication. It can be a long and tedious process but if carried out effectively, becomes the backbone of the clinical management. Not only doctors but nurses and other staff members can also facilitate the patient if he or she is uncomfortable and unable to share a proper history.

Avoiding and resolving conflict in difficult situations:

As discussed above, there are a thousand things that can go wrong while a patient is visiting a hospital. The staff of the healthcare setups should have a clear understanding of the problems the patients may face. The problems can be of different types e.g. administrative, environmental, behavioral, etc.

Some patients don't like waiting too long. Waiting conditions can make certain patients angry and frustrated. Some patients may be too old and fatigued to wait that long. Sooner or later such patients act out and express aggression. The staff should make sure that they figure out ways to communicate with such patients, ask them what can make them comfortable, reassure them and try their best to ease them out.

Sometimes, "breaking bad news" can lead to difficult situations. Death of loved ones can make people show a variety of emotions. Passing through stages of grief, relatives of the patients can blame the healthcare staff if they have not been appropriately informed and counselled about the patient's condition. Communicating "proactively" in this case is essential.

Ensuring the safety of transitioning of patient care:

Transitioning of patient care from one healthcare setting to another is critical for patients and families. Transitioning can be of different types. One type of transitioning is from acute care to home e.g. *going home after a road traffic accident with multiple injuries and fractures.* Another type ranges from wellness to chronic management of the disease, e.g. *lifestyle modification and rehabilitation after recovering from acute ischemic stroke.* During both the types, multiple opportunities are present, where important aspects of healthcare communication can be missed.

One can always relate to it, especially if one has had such an experience. Whether the transitioning is one's own as a patient or a loved one's caregiver, one may agree that such times cause a significant degree of panic and anxiety owing to a heightened concern about what to will happen next. From the healthcare communication angle, these are exactly the situations where transferring and ensuring the understanding of the key information about patient care should be made possible.

Why communication is important in social health care?

A patient and his family are required to absorb a lot of health information, and especially learning about new medications is particularly not less than a challenge. In addition, clinical symptoms, follow-up care and visits, requirement of a possible physical therapy and social determinants of health also influence the patient's recovery, significantly. Health literacy and social determinants of health are important issues affecting patient recovery after a stay in the hospital. Also, changes in refunding of payments can have an impact on the length of stay, which may shorten. This can also affect the patients by not giving them enough time and opportunity to engulf the information about the plan of care moving on to the next setting or home.

a) Planning a discharge from the health facilities:

Discharging the patient or shifting the care of the patient to their primary care givers is always a challenge, especially getting discharged after a prolonged stay in hospital. Planning a discharge is generally a complex procedure. Care staff should be able to summarize and communicate significant information which is tailored according to functional status of the patient, their preferences and follow-up care.

It often happens in the hospitals that due to the busy nature of the wards, doctors may discharge the patients "in haste". They rush through by not sharing important instructions regarding the discharge and instructions. Sometimes, they only rely on the other healthcare staff for complete information sharing, what seems to be their own primary responsibility. However, they may not do this deliberately This hasty communication does not leave a positive impact on the patient, rather a negative one. It can severely affect a patient's understanding of his disease and recovery prospects and can lead to noncompliance with the care plan. A lot of patients if asked, will respond by saying that they don't comprehend the information shared with them at the time of discharges. These are seemingly non-clinical issues but they have a profound impact. This transition from the hospital care to the homecare can lead to many voids in the patient care, even when the patients are always more comfortable in the home environment than at the hospital.

b) <u>Smoothening out the transitioning of patients from hospital to homecare:</u>

A lot of health systems have engineered and sustained specifically targeted workflows to prepare the patients for safe transitions from hospital to home. These workflows are specialized communication channels that help in improving the methods of communications between patient and hospital's care team during this transitional journey.

The main purpose of such communication channels is the establishment of two types of communication:

1. Conduction of rounds prior to discharge
2. Outreach calls after the discharge to catch up with the patient's progress and keep track of patient's recovery.

1. <u>Rounding prior to transition to ensure optimum patient care:</u>

This round mainly consists of a final review of the discharge plan which is often "personalized". The focus remains on:

- Homecare requirements
- Monitoring of patient's signs and symptoms
- Availability of reliable and durable medical equipment
- Patient safety information
- Transportation
- Care instructions
- Follow-up appointments

To make these rounds purposeful, healthcare staff including the clinicians and nurses should have a sympathetic communication with the patients that do not feel tightly scripted. This important interaction should not be rushed, rather relaxed and not hurried.

Verbal communication is very important in this scenario: e.g., asking for permission to sit down beside the patients and pulling the chair close to the bed can have a lasting effect on the patient. It has been proven by studies that patients feel more connected to the doctors when they sit with them rather keep standing when they visit them. This also gives the patient the perception of the doctor having spent more time with them. Therefore, patient's sentiments about their health providers very much depend on the quality of the communication they have with them, because patients generally remember the kindness, attention and respect they received from them.

2. <u>Outreach calls after the discharge to catch up with the patient's progress and keep track of patient's recovery</u>

To ensure that the patients stay committed to the designated plan for recovery, healthcare staff should follow up with their patients. They must provide the patients the opportunity to ask for assistance and guidance. It is vital for the health systems to develop a reliable, effective and consistent outreach programs post-discharge. This may include visits and automated phone calls. These post-discharge calls confirm that the transition place is intact and is being followed efficiently. Assessment about patient's and care givers' understanding and need of further assistance is made.

Patients should also be educated about receiving the automated calls during the rounds. Before discharging, a nurse should be available to talk to them if they reach out with any queries related to the outreach program. This will impart a personal touch to the process of automated calls.

The patients have a greater chance at equipping themselves by this proactive method of communication, i.e. patient engagement following discharge. Overall, this leads to beneficial patient outcomes, healthy patient satisfaction and less number of readmissions.

Effective healthcare communication: what does the research say?

A retrospective study was conducted at a healthcare setup located in the U.S. in which the effectiveness of these specialized communication strategies implemented on patients was gauged: more than 7% patients remained confused regarding their health plan after discharge as they didn't receive their care round prior to discharge, as compared to 4% who complained of confusion even after receiving the detailed, final visit. Therefore, the likelihood of confusion increased when the final, pre-discharge round had not taken place.

Another study done by the same healthcare facility that analyzed the post-discharge outreach, more than 50% patients who completed the calls and responded to it, seldom needed readmission.

Communication in healthcare: improving patients' healthcare experience

a) Developing patient trust:

A patient's trust on the healthcare system develops through clinical encounters and sometimes strictly nonclinical "microencounters" with the healthcare staff. Both medical and non-medical factors play an important role and can ultimately affect their health outcomes. A good communication between the healthcare staff and patient is important to build a relationship based on trust. Patients are unlikely to share vital and critical information related to their ailments when they don't trust the health system.

Healthcare staff can build trust of the patients by providing personalized and timely information to them. They can ensure that they familiarize the patients with the opportunities available to them for acquiring better health care for themselves.

To summarize, a trip to the hospital is discomforting for patients and their families. The desire to know about their illnesses and having an exhaustive list of questions in their minds makes them apprehensive and overwhelmed. These feelings compounded by the lingering fear of loss of functionality – they can feel that they are losing control. The variety of negative psychological emotions can have an overall negative influence on their disease outcomes.

Healthcare teams have a shot at the opportunity to maintain the patient's dignity in these situations of adverse outcomes and dubiety through effective "patient-centered" communication. Communication channels must be able to help the patients and have a far-reaching effect on them even beyond the premises of the healthcare facility. Good communication is part and parcel of today's complex, personalized and dignified healthcare and the patients certainly deserve nothing short of it.

b) Improving patient satisfaction:

The basic elements of patient satisfaction are based are:

Pateint Expectations	• Giving patients ample opportunity to narate their story comfortably and the feeling of being "listened to"
Healthcare (clinical) team	• The patient's first worry about the healthcare system is the clinician they will be entrusted to. So, if they are satisfied with the clinician, they also value the healthcare team that clinician is a part of
Effective communication	• It involves listening to the problems of the patients, patiently, explaining the health information clearly, show empathy, relate with the patient's experience and lay out the viable treatment options available.
Patient dignity	• Patients treated with respect and are given the opportunity to get involved in their own healthcare decisions show and report more satisfaction
Inititation of referrals	• It brings the patients great satisfaction when their team decides to refer them on their own because it makes them feel relieved of this responsibility
Decision-making	• When importance is given to patients' social and psychological wellbeing as much as physical wellbeing, patients acknowledge it and it increases their satisfaction
Patient control	• Patient satisfaction increases when patients are motivated and encouraged to express their thoughts, concerns, ideas and expectations
Length of the time spent	• Improvement in patient satisfaction takes place as the length of the visit increases
Continuous care	• Reception of continuing care from the same healthcare team brings the patients much needed satisfaction in times of physical and mental dstress.

c) Ensuring patient safety:

It has been estimated that approximately one-third of untoward events are attributable to either human errors or system errors. After a decade of research conducted from 1995-2005, it has been concluded that inadequate team communication is the basic cause for about 66% of total medical errors during the period specified. This implies that the when healthcare team partners do not communicate directly and efficiently, patient care is bound to suffers, one way or the other.

Furthermore, chances of vulnerability to medical errors elevate when healthcare team members are stressed out, facing challenging and high-risk situations, and when proper communication Is not being taken place clearly.

d) Maintaining team satisfaction:

i. Importance of team satisfaction and why?

The quality of healthcare communication between the team members directly affects these three things: quality of professional relationships of healthcare staff, their job satisfaction and patient safety. Evidence from research has shown that when everyone among the staff members is well-informed about rights and responsibilities and well-communicated about patient care, significant decline in health staff turnover has been observed. In addition, better job satisfaction results as a culture of mutual respect and support is promoted. Larson and Yao, two researchers, have discovered a direct correlation between level of clinician's satisfaction and ability to build rapport and expression of care and warmth with patients.

ii. Factors contributing to healthcare team satisfaction:

Feeling valued, respected, understood, listened too, supported in terms of administrative tasks and interpersonal relationships; and having clarity of job description, equality of work and fairness in compensation are some of the factors contributing to the satisfaction of the healthcare team.

Risk of malpractice – how is it related to ineffective communication in healthcare?

Huntington and Kuhn reported that the ultimate "root cause" of malpractice claims is actually a communication gap between a physician and a patient. Previously, studies reviewing plaintiff depositions concluded that 71% of malpractice claims initially began as a result of problems in physician's and patient's "relationship". Looking more closely, it was found that most patients who were involved in litigation with their physicians often had a perception that physician are "not sincere or caring". Same researchers concluded that in malpractice cases, 25% plaintiffs explained the reason for litigation as "poor information delivery", with 13% think that the reason is "the physicians didn't listen well".

Importance of communication in healthcare: TIDBITS

- It has been pointed out by various studies that communication skills of health staff, the patient's ability to follow the medical advice, self-manage a chronic disease switch to a preventive lifestyle: are all positively co-related

- Moreover, the doctor's explanation of the problem, ability to listen and empathize can have a far-reaching impact on every kind of health outcomes whether psychological or physical, as well as patient care and satisfaction

- Moving further, communication between the healthcare staff, especially belonging to the same team, affect the environment of the healthcare facility, quality of professional relationships, job satisfaction of the staff and patient care.

- Every member of the healthcare team organizes and conducts thousands of patient interactions throughout their careers. It is always advisable to "communicate" well because whatever has to be done, has to be done in the right way.

- The importance of "communication training" for the healthcare staff, especially clinicians and nurses, cannot be emphasized enough. As with other healthcare procedures, communication skills can also be learned, improvements can be made along the way, however, it needs commitment and practice.

- There is astounding evidence which relates inadequate clinician-patient communication with increased risk of malpractice and negligence, treatment noncompliance, dissatisfaction, and unattained health goals. Therefore, there is no denying how much necessary acquiring skills for effective communication is.

CHAPTER 4

How to communicate effectively in healthcare?

"Good communication is a bridge between confusion and clarity" – Nat Turner

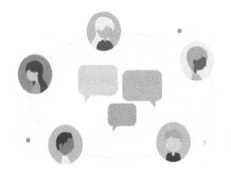

What Is Effective Communication in Healthcare?

"Effective communication" refers to *"direct and open communication between the healthcare professionals: clear, appropriately timed, relevant and discrete".* The importance of such kind of communication has already been discussed and one cannot ignore it because it is required to make accurate diagnoses of diseases, promises provision of appropriate treatments and ensures patient's understanding of his condition.

Effective communication between the healthcare professionals can be of two types:

  a. Within the hospital: **intrahospital communication**
  b. Within two different hospitals: **interhospital communication**

Interhospital communication play an important part in patient protection, cost-effectiveness and enhanced efficacy of routine projects. For patients, this communication saves their time and their lives too: due to increased access for the other hospital to their detailed present and past medical histories with reduced chances of making medical errors.

Comparing interhospital and intrahospital communications

Both these types of institutional communication methods in use, are critical to patient's safety, health and recovery. Let us anlyze both of them.

a) Interhospital:

"Interhospital" (**inter-** meaning *between*) communication revolves around sharing of relevant healthcare information at multiple sites or institutions. These institutes can be a part of the same organization or separate facilities. It is customary to maintain excellent communication between the two, to make the overall healthcare experience better for the patients.

Often, hospitals face certain obstacles in this type of effective communication. Center for Health Information and Decision Systems (CHIDS) conducted a study and concluded that ineffective interhospital communication channels can lead to whopping monetary losses to healthcare industry, amounting to more than $12 billion per annum. The reason costs are driven up due to inadequate communication is that health institutions are prevented from accessing the patients' medical record which leads to duplication of clinical investigations and second opinions that would not be needed, otherwise.

b) Intrahospital

"Intrahospital" (**intra-** meaning *within*) communication, that occurs between the personnel of the same hospital, cannot be perfect everywhere. Mostly, it refers to any information shared within an institute e.g. requesting further investigations, synchronizing room changes, scheduling surgical and medical procedures or something as simple as lining up the clinical appointments, etc. When the information is not being shared and discussed between staff and patients, this may lead to decreased efficiency of the whole system. As a result, there can be penalties in the form of extraneous costs and detriment to patient safety. Other consequences include unusual delays in patient record-keeping, poor procedural coordination and even medical negligence.

A few tips and tricks for open, effective communication in healthcare:

Simple, clear language should be used at all times, whatever the circumstances	The consultation style should be pliable and modifiable	Active listening should be practiced	Empathetic atitude should be demonstrated

Develop a habit of engaging patients in effective dialogue	Always be careful about the body language while communicating (non-verbal communication)	Always keep colleagues and other members of the health team in the "communication loop

Tips and tricks for open healthcare communication

"If you talk to a man in a language he understands, that goes to his head. If you talk to him in his language, that goes to his heart" - Nelson Mandela

Effective communication of information pertaining to healthcare permits the patients and caregivers to partake in the affairs of their healthcare as partners. It has been known to solidify the patient compliance to treatment and self-management. It should be further implied that the significance of patient and healthcare staff's communication is stretched out far beyond the healthcare facility setting.

So, while summarizing, it will be okay to say that there are seven strategies you can adopt to communicate effectively:

1. Clarify your objective

2. Structure your thinking

3. Manage your time

4. Find common ground

5. Move beyond argument

6. Summarize often

7. Use visuals

Types of communication skills and how they interrelate

There are three broad categories of skills that need to be learnt by and trained in, by all healthcare professionals summarized in the image below.

Content skills

- What is being communicated by the healthcare professionals? the questions and responses, information they gather and give, the treatments they discuss.

Process skills

- How they do it? the ways in which they communicate with patients, how they note down history or providing information, verbal and non-verbal skills, how they develop the relationship with the patient, the way in which they organise and structure communication.

Perceptual skills

- What they are thinking and feeling – their internal decisionmaking, clinical-reasoning and problem-solving skills; their attitudes; their
- Personal capacities for compassion, kindness, mindfulness, empathy, integrity, respect and flexibility; their awareness of feelings about the patient, about the illness and about other concerning issues; awareness of their own self-concept and confidence, of their own biases and distractions.

Basic skill needed by healthcare workers for effective communication

It is important to emphasize that these skills are fantastically linked and cannot be expected to exist alone. Attention must be paid to all three types of skills. Communication process skills and the deep entanglement of these three types of skills receive very less attention in medical curricula.

Using basic communication in certain situations:

a) Patient-centered communication:

It is a common occurrence in healthcare setups that doctors or nurses have to break bad news to the patients or their family members. As herculean as this task may be, it can be performed effortlessly through effective communication. But it needs refined communication skills, patience and the most important skill: empathy for everyone involved. Although there are various methods for delivering undesirable news to the patient, the successful ones are always "patient-centered".

Without empathy and well-developed communication skills, the doctors and nurses will not be able to provide dedicated care to the patients.

Regardless of the healthcare provider, patient-centered communication is very important contributing factor to impart quality patient care. Most medical schools and universities all over the world now offer training courses in communication. Some medical universities integrate content related to learning of communication skills in their curriculum.

All medical license exams (USMLE, PLAB, AMC) and even Occupational English Test (OET) for healthcare practitioners needs communication skills to be demonstrated. Patient-centered communication methodologies are also taught in nursing schools religiously, however, like other new skills, student fail to integrate them into clinical practice. These skills need to be revised, rehearsed, modeled and reinforced time and again, under faculty supervision.

b) Delivering bad news:

One of the most difficult situations to have faced in the repertoire of any healthcare practitioner's communication skills is art of "breaking bad news" to the patients and their families. Many doctors and nurses mistakenly believe that being able to break bad news is a skill important only for clinicians employed in end-of-life care. In end-of-life-care setups, one isy expected to announce end of treatment citing it "unsuccessful" without providing any option for relief: "the death is most certainly imminent". However, every healthcare provider must know how to deliver bad news to different tiers of population on different levels, at different times.

Let us dive a little deeper into the ocean of "bad news". Bad news can be defined as

"any news or information that affects a person's view of the future in a negative manner"

The doctor or nurse have no authority to judge about what kind of news should sound "bad" to the patient. They should be familiar with any type of information that can potentially change an individual's entire scope of themselves, their reality or their future. For doctors, it is a responsibility on their shoulders, diagnosing a life-ending disease. However, "breaking bad news" does not only limit to informing about imminent death, it also involves communicating the news to the patients and families:

- When a new diagnosis has been made
- If a chronic illness has deteriorated

- Or if conventional pharmacological and non-pharmacologic interventions have not been proven fruitful and a new treatment plan needs to be devised.

Breaking bad news is a multifarious task and needs cautious efforts to manage it brilliantly. Many aspects of this kind of communication are fairly foreseeable, especially if the patient is already under nursing and consultant care in specialty practice.

The doctors can make a mental strategy for delivering bad news. Not only this but dealing with the emotions of patients and their families and inform them about further plan of care can be planned efficiently. But the only prerequisite is: establishment of a reasonable degree of relationship with the patient. This communication should take place with utmost concern for the receivers of the bad news. A template can be used to follow in such situations while conveying bad news that will assist in instilling and assuring quality and "human emotions" into this challenging process....

A great magnitude of professionalism, stamina and patience is required for delivering bad news uneventfully. This process is complex and requires the doctors and nurses:

- To find appropriate "kind" words
- To use understandable terminology (no complex medical jargon)
- To assess the reaction of the patient and family and the degree of agony that whole conversation is inducing.
- To tailor the information as the doctor responds to third step, the assessment process.
- Lastly, to steer the conversation from the "bad news" to the "future plans" (*focusing on the solution, not the problem*) with hope, realism and optimism.

There are many accepted methods of breaking bad news which include:

- "Conventional method of structured listening": the patient has a great deal of idea about his illness and wants to know more
- "Giving concise, relevant information in appropriate amounts": don't let the patient feel overwhelmed
- Reacting to the news
- And checking for patient's understanding

The SPIKES Protocol

"SPIKES" is an acronym which stands for:

S	Setting up
P	Perception
I	Invitation
K	Knowledge
E	Emotions with Empathy
S	Strategy/Summary

This approach for delivering bad news to the patients, was developed and designed by Walter Baile and his peers at the University of Texas (MD Anderson Cancer Center, Houston, Texas).

Steps to follow for breaking bad news:

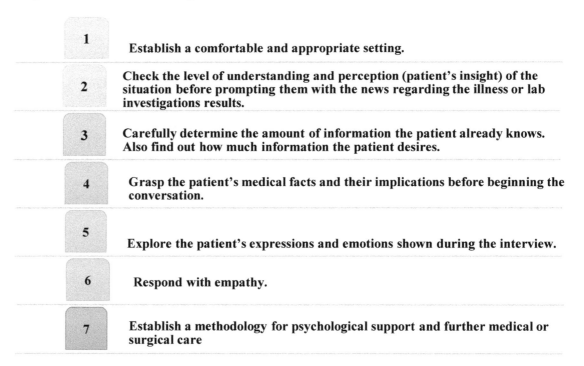

1	Establish a comfortable and appropriate setting.
2	Check the level of understanding and perception (patient's insight) of the situation before prompting them with the news regarding the illness or lab investigations results.
3	Carefully determine the amount of information the patient already knows. Also find out how much information the patient desires.
4	Grasp the patient's medical facts and their implications before beginning the conversation.
5	Explore the patient's expressions and emotions shown during the interview.
6	Respond with empathy.
7	Establish a methodology for psychological support and further medical or surgical care

Let us view each step in detail:

Steps	Description
Setting Up	The first step in SPIKES protocol is setting up the interview. It includes the following: • Be well-prepared about the information to be shared by rehearsing the dialogue in mind • The appropriate vocabulary to be used can also be reviewed prior to the conversation begins • Review notes, discuss likely implications of the news with team members and knowledge of the specific care plan • Novice doctors and nurses should pay attention to this step for more confident and excellent communication • A united, strong and uniform message from the whole team is essential • Pay attention to the physical space and the way in which the news will be shared. A wrong physical setting can lead to an unsuccessful interaction • Preferred body language: maintain an open posture, sit while speaking and maintain eye contact • Provide privacy even if in a busy clinic: quiet space during dialogue. • Ask the patient to mute their personal communication devices can also lessen the chances of interruption and minimize distraction • Be confident, eliminate the nervousness • Place your feet flat on the floor, put your ankles together and keep hands and eyes in lap (neutral position) • Maintain eye contact to show your attentiveness
Perception	Patient's perception of the bad news depends on how it is conveyed to the patient. • Fully assess what the patients and family know about the test results, what will it mean to them relative to the illness and the amount of information they desire • Build a reasonable degree of relationship with the patient by following through a workup and diagnostic workup or management of chronic illness, to assess patient's perception • Empathic skills will always help. Response of the patient will guide the next step • Interpret if the patient has any misconception about the seriousness of the illness and doesn't have any unrealistic expectations, wishful thinking, does not omit crucial medical information • Do not shatter the "denial" phase, if there, as it helps as a good coping mechanism • Provide informed consent for any further testing and management
Invitation	• After gauging the extent of information required by the patient, ask for permission to share the details regarding current news • In addition, ask for permission regarding sharing the news with their family

Knowledge	• *Fire a Warning Shot*: take the first step and give them a heads up about the incoming news not being very good.
	• Begin the news-sharing with phrases such as:
	  - *"Unfortunately the news which I am about to share with you is not good"*
	  - *"I am really sorry to tell you"*
	  - *"Things are not going ahead the way we had hoped them to"*
	  - *"I am afraid the news which I am about to give you is not what you may like at this moment"*
	  - *"You may not like the news which I am about to share with you but I am really sorry"*
	This helps the patients and their family to get themselves emotionally prepared for the information that will follow.
	• The doctor should sound like the patient's solicitor rather than a third party divulging devastating information.
	• The news must be presented keeping in mind the pre-assessed parameters of patient's knowledge, compliance and desires for information disclosure
	• Don't use technical jargon, show them examples like lab investigations, results from radiology: to clear their abstract concepts
	• Do the whole process really slowly for everyone to understand.
	• Choose words carefully, especially if the news tells about poor prognosis
	• **News involving cancer diagnosis**: doctor should be skillfully prepared for meeting the information needs of the patients. The content, doctor's expertise and relevant details are all very significant in this case.

Empathy	• The doctor should express an understanding of the patient's condition and emotional situation and should demonstrate empathy and respect. • *Be patient with the patient.* They can display a spectrum of emotions and reaction, from silence to sobbing to dramatic crying. This awkward situation can only be dealt with empathy and a kind response.
Plan a strategy for the future	• Prepare the patient for participation in their own future management plans. This will reduce the overall distress irrespective of the stage of illness. • Ensure their understanding of the information given to them • Ask the patient before discussing further management plan if they are prepared to have this discussion. Ask for frequent clarifications during this conversation. • In the end, always leave with a clear plan regarding further treatment. Arrange for more lab investigation if required and make them understand about the way those results will be communicated with them

Refining communication skills

Learning communication skill had both cognitive and experiential components. Skill such as "breaking bad news" for healthcare workers needs more experiential learning rather than just theoretical and the use of didactic methodology is also important while learning it. Ideally it should be taught as a "psychomotor" skill and ample opportunity must be provided during the training phases to "practice" it in a controlled environment, followed by allowing them to implement those skills in a clinical environment.

Barriers in healthcare communication:

Hindrance and some potential barriers in the way of direct, effective communication between the nursing staff and patients can be due to:

- A plethora of demands and challenges
- Time constraint
- Burden of the work
- Considerable lack of privacy
- Environment with overwhelming background noise

Some factors that affect the ability of the patients to communicate effectively are:

- Their health conditions
- Their medications
- Language barrier
- Cultural and social barriers
- Pain and discomfort
- Anxiety
- Long waiting times

"Communication is power. Those who have mastered its effective use can change their own experience of the world and the world's experience of them. All behaviors and feelings find their original roots in some form of communication" – Tony Robbins

Overcoming barriers in health communication:

After identifying and understanding the barriers in health communication, the next step should be to try an overcome those barriers.

Ask your patient to tell you all the details related to his illness - "talk like a parrot". Medical memory can help overcome communication challenges.

Be at the same seating level as the patient.

Maintain appropriate eye contact, be visual to the patient

Record all the patient visits

Always ensure the use of use easy-to-understand language and not medical jargon

Learn to listen and understand, not to listen and just reply

Overcoming barriers in healthcare communication

Significance of communication in healthcare:

Hospitals and healthcare institutes should ensure proper patient care and to make that possible, they should look past formulating a diagnosis and performing a procedure. Understanding that communication is a pivotal component in nearly every step of healthcare process, is the only way forward towards excellence. No matter if it is just a clinic sharing patient information word for word with another health facility, or a cohort of doctors, nurses, consultants and other staff at a hospital engaged in discussions regarding the treatment of current patients and patients expected to come. Direct, concise and effective communication will always be the ultimate need of every health system.

Institutes with strong institutional communication methodologies help patients recover earlier while those that don't can adversely affect the patient's well-being. It is the need of the hour that the healthcare professionals and institutions recognize how survival largely depends on communication.

Better communication: why is it advantageous?

According to a research published in "Fierce Healthcare", unsatisfactory communication has been recognized as a causative factor that resulted in 1,744 patient deaths and more than $1.7 billion in the cost of malpractice fine all over the U.S in half a decade. It is evident enough that better communication methods are important for both the patients and healthcare staff.

Healthcare communication: a focus on patient safety:

Patient safety is the most important motivating factor that drives health organizations to develop effective communication strategies, considering that very often, the leading cause of in-hospital deaths is inadequate or faulty communication methods. A 2006 study published in *"Clinical Biochemist Review"* summarizes that while reviewing in-hospital deaths retrospectively, a humungous number of 14,000 deaths could be traced down to have occurred mainly due to "grave communication errors". Moreover, the results implied that deaths due to lack of communication are believed to occur two-times more frequently than substandard or poor clinical skill.

While the repercussions of having poor communication methods in a health facility are harsh, this is nothing that cannot be fixed. Rather it is not that hard once there is realization and room for improvement. In other words, such patient deaths due to these notorious communication errors are entirely preventable. This alone suffices to explain what good communication means for patient safety.

Patient safety: common methods for effective communication

Many methods of communication exist for healthcare institutes and all the administrative as well as clinical staff must be well-trained to utilize it proficiently. Failure of even one type of method is enough to expose patients to considerable risk. For example, a minute typographical error during printing can have disastrous outcomes especially if incorrect dosages were printed. Similarly, incomplete details may prevent a doctor from knowing about severe life-threatening allergic reaction a patient may suffer from.

The first step towards ensuring fluent communication between hospital staff is understanding how these "standard" communication methods work – for the sake of patients' life and staff's professional careers.

Some of the most common methods for "effective communication" in healthcare are:

1. <u>Coordination with the hospital leadership</u>:

Both public and private hospitals are funded as both are essentially "businesses" which are required to operate as such. The hospital management team members and leaders should frequently stay in touch doctors, nursing staff, administrative staff and patients. They should not only supervise administrative tasks but also play pivotal role in personalized healthcare plan for patients. Channels of communication should always remain open with all the people around them in order to provide effective healthcare and also expedite interdepartmental and interhospital sharing of information.

2. <u>Using telemedicine</u>:

Telemedicine has been in practice for many years now but professionals in healthcare have embraced telemedicine to be an important part of health communication since the COVID-19 pandemic hit the world. according to "American Telemedicine Association", a wide variety of internet-based applications and technologies are being used nowadays to communicate with patients remotely (online). Such technological tools play an integral role in health communication.

Hospitals and other organizations concerned with patient health make use of central or institutional web networks or "intranets" to run effective communication processes. This has made the record sharing and interdepartmental information flow much swifter. Previously, innumerable printed files with lots of paperwork were required for patient data recording and information sharing. Now, files and memorandums are routinely shared electronically within the institute and between two different organizations.

Telemedicine is a step ahead as it permits patients to access medical care and consultation from the comfortable environment of their own homes. It utilizes the state-of-the-art tools for communication which allow the healthcare providers to discuss health concerns with their patients via video call, thus, bypassing the need for visiting the doctor's office. Overall, a smooth, seamless experience for everyone. However, by far, the most beneficial aspect is the dramatically reduced cost for both the participants.

Effective healthcare communication - outcomes

A clinician conducts many patient interviews throughout a typical career, as much as 150,000 interviews. If patient interview is considered as a healthcare procedure, it is the most commonly used procedure that any clinician use. But for some reason, training for excelling at health communication for clinicians and other healthcare professionals has never received any credible attention historically if we compare it with a skill related to any common medical or surgical procedure.

1. Diagnostic Accuracy

The formulation of the clinical diagnosis starts when the clinician beings the history-taking part of the patient interview. However, research says that still many patients feel that they haven't been listened well r given the time to tell their complete story. This can be due to interruptions during their interview, which can compromise the accuracy of their diagnostic process. Therefore, incomplete histories lead to incomplete record of data and hence, faulty clinical decisions. Moreover, the interruptions can make the patients believe that whatever they have to say is not important and they become hesitant to share more information. The bottom line is that when interruptions occur, it deters the patients from sharing essential information and it and it damages the doctor-patient relationship.

2. Adherence

Adherence, also called compliance, is defined as the measure of how much the patient follows doctor's recommendations which he agreed upon or changes his behavior corresponding to the doctor's advice. Certainly, the problem of non-adherence or non-compliance are very well-known to healthcare providers. For example, a Health Care Quality Survey was conducted by "Commonwealth fund" observed that 25% of Americans report non-adherence to clinician's health and treatment advice. The reasons were:

- 39% didn't agree with the doctor's advice and recommendations
- 27% were worried about costs if they comply
- For 25%, the instructions were not explained enough and were difficult to follow
- 20% believed that the doctor's recommendations were contrary to what their personal beliefs are
- Lastly, 7% stated the reason of noncompliance as not having any knowledge about what needs to be done

3. Safe and effective transmission of patient data

Patient information is shared safely and securely via inter-and intrahospital communication channels. Millions of dollars need to be additionally spent if the health information is not received in time by the concerned staff. Medical history is created through the use of patient data for the provision of appropriate care. When patient data aren't shared between departments or other health organizations, there may be higher practice error chances and cost increment.

4. Effective sharing of research findings

For improvement in therapeutic procedures and communication methodologies, the healthcare industry hugely depends on researches. However, some private (third-party researchers) belonging to private or pharmaceutical companies show reluctance in sharing their results with health providers due to competition in their industries. If the results of latest researches are not accessed or analyzed, it can lead to delayed medical advancement, funds wastage and negative effect on health outcomes, as stated by an article in Forbes. For evolution of therapeutic techniques, healthcare workers must design and introduce health communication systems that can quickly collaborate with researchers, both within an organization or between different organizations.

5. Effective collaboration while working with colleagues

Intrahospital communication is greatly dependent on collaboration among healthcare team members or "colleagues". These include information sharing between patients, doctors, nurses, lab technologists, and other staff, all need to be in line with the coordination in order to create a smoothly operating system. Collaboration among colleagues also includes ensuring that correct entry of patient data into the hospital database which is shared with all the staff members. Inadequate interdepartmental communication can result in erroneous database entries, which pose the greatest risk to patient safety.

Effective communication: tidbits

In this age of information overload, the attention span of our people is short due to non-stop distractions around. In these circumstances, it is becoming increasingly important to have effective communication to provide healthcare efficiently. Many a times, just talking to the patient for a while before starting to discuss their health condition with them, asking a few extra questions, and giving information and educational brochures can bring the feeling of a "different experience". And in the light of this interaction, patients begin to view their relationship with doctors in a different light and it positively affects how they talk to their friends and family about their doctors.

Sources:

Rosenzweig MQ. Breaking bad news: a guide for effective and empathetic communication. Nurse Pract. 2012 Feb 12;37(2):1-4. doi: 10.1097/01.NPR.0000408626.24599.9e. PMID: 22252021; PMCID: PMC5578619.

CHAPTER 5

Ethical and legal aspects of communication in healthcare

"Effective health communication is the art and technique of informing, influencing, and motivating individuals, institutions, and large public audiences about important health issues based on sound scientific and ethical considerations"

(Tufts University Student Services, 2006)

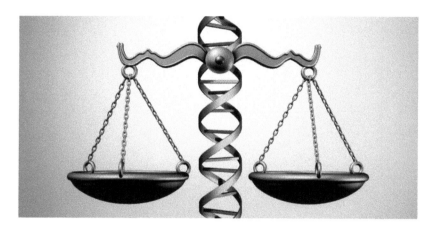

Authentic and sensitive communication of healthcare information is pivotal to providing good quality patient care, whether the patient need pain management in a pain clinic, surgical procedure in operating theatre or other health interventions in any other setting. However, health information i.e. data of the patient is sensitive and may cause embarrassment if it "leaks out" or falls into the wrong hands. Ethical standards of medicine maintain that this is the obligation of the doctors to safeguard the patient's confidential information. But there are many threats always hovering around the confidential information, more so in this age of instant communication through the use of emails, internet and facsimile.

Nowadays, medical information can be transmitted widely, instantaneously and effortlessly, which provides a tremendous opportunity to provide quality health care by stating complete, correct and timely patient data to the practitioners when needed. But this rapid dissemination of medical data has its downside. For example, traditional paper charts if available to a "some" care providers, an e-medical record is accessible to hundreds and thousands of people.

There are ample chances of potential damage if that information is inaccurate, such an ill-advised communication can lead to disastrous consequences. Given the circumstances, it was never more important for healthcare workers to acquire vestigial knowledge about legal and ethical implications of healthcare communication.

Importance of communication in medical settings has always been taken for granted but it is never too late to set your priorities right.

Legal issues in health communication

The three most important legal issues pertaining to healthcare communication are:

1. Confidentiality breach/privacy breach
2. Informed consent
3. Defamation

A delicate balance between sharing healthcare information and guarding sensitive patient information needs to be achieved.

1. Confidentiality breach/privacy breach:

Consider this scenario:

Mr. Albert is a patient visiting a rheumatology clinic of a medical center for chronic back pain. On history-taking, Dr. Stephen got to know about his history of intravenous drug abuse. An ELISA screening was requested that came out to be Hepatitis C positive. He notified this positive result to the local health department and was asked to send the copy of email of patient's clinic visit. Mr. Albert sued the doctor for privacy invasion and confidentiality breach when he learned about this incident.

One of the most important ideas deeply engraved into the modern Western philosophy is the idea of **"personal privacy"** or **"personal autonomy"**. It can be defined as

"the priority of an individual as different or distinct from the welfare of his/her social group". Or in my own words, "pride in individuality."

The concept originated during the Renaissance period when personal rights and responsibilities started to gain important in the society. The **"right to privacy"** can be defined as

"the right to be left independent and alone to perform personal affairs without unreasonable interference from the government, any organization or any other person, as long as one's conduct is not unlawful or indecent"

Confidentiality is just another subset of privacy dealing with communication of patient information. Therefore, it is the right of "personal autonomy" which encompasses all the other rights, i.e. right to control dissemination of personal information. Both Hippocratic Oath and American Medical Association (AMA) Code of Ethics explain medical confidentiality. AMA defines it as:

"A physician shall respect the rights of patients, of colleagues and of other health professionals, and shall safeguard patient confidences within the constraints of the law"

The confidentiality of the doctor-patient relationship is the basis on which the trust is established the trust, which is vital to providing effective patient care. When the sanctity of this relationship is not maintained, and information is shared inappropriately, the trust gets eroded. The constitutions of many countries do not contain any legal provision ensuring the right of personal privacy. However, privacy breach or invasion is a well-known tort (legal cause of action) or crime and the law certainly provides legal solution for compensation.

Despite of the fact that law and medical ethics recognize that rights to personal privacy, there exist some ambiguous and confusing federal laws and court verdicts that renders it impossible to be liable to full protection.

Doctors always abide by the ethical and legal restrictions on them about disclosing confidential patient information, many exceptions exist. This allows large amounts of patient information to be shared: "the only reasonable expectation of privacy is no expectation of privacy at all". This especially holds true today in this era of fast communication. The information sharing is vital to patient care and needs frequent movement along with the patient, as he gets transferred to other facilities. In this case, e-medical records really make things easier. With a single click on a computer, authentic, complete and timely information makes its way to the other side of the country or world. This increases efficiency and decrease costs. Analysis of electronic patient data can help in improving standard of medical practice and use of health care resources.

The ease of information-sharing comes with a price: the sacrifice of patient privacy to variable extents. Information can be shared inappropriately as it is displayed on a computer screen and anyone who passes by can observe it. Health insurance officers, public health authorities' representatives, researchers, peer reviewers and quality assurance officers, all have rights to access patient information. Consent to release information is often acquired by simple signature from the patient on the treatment form, no separate paperwork for consent acquisition is done. In many parts of the world, the patients are not eve told that they are signing consent when they put initials on the treatment form. So, there is always chances of unauthorized data release.

2. Informed consent:

Read this scenario:

Dr. Yamaha is a neurologist in a clinic which is administered by a local health organization. He believes that patient Ms. Mariah would benefit from a hand-held device called Vagal Nerve Stimulator for her crippling, resistant, chronic migraine headaches but her health plan does not cover the purchase of such a device. He also discusses this with her during the next visit but also informs her about her insurance plan's inability to cover for that device. Dr. Yamaha's employment contract with the health organization does not allow him from telling her about the procedures or treatments not covered by their health plan. When the organization learns about his suggestion of such a device as a treatment plan, it dropped him from its panel.

"Personal autonomy" means a person's (or patient's) "consent" given ahead of any type of evaluation and treatment suggested by the physician. In 1914, Justice Cardozo said these famous words

"Every human being of adult years and sound mind has a right to determine what shall be done with his own body; a surgeon who performs an operation without his patient's consent commits an assault for which he is liable in damages. This is true except in cases of emergency, where the patient is unconscious and where it is necessary to operate before consent can be obtained"

These century-old words are coming true today. The doctors are now under a strict obligation, (except in limited emergency situations) to seek consent and that too informed consent, even before examination and beginning of treatment. Informed consent can be defined as

"giving the patient complete, accurate and relevant information about the expected treatment including all the risks, benefits, and alternatives."

To test this, the favorable question to ask is "what a reasonable person need to be told to want to give an informed consent and take further decisions?". In many parts of the world there are "informed consent statutes" which determines and guides about the type of information to be disclosed to the patient in order to give informed consent"

Despite its essentiality, informed consent in not always effective. According to a decades-old survey, doctors hand out inadequate and unclear information to the patients which can negatively influence their decisions. There is obviously a conflict in some situation: on one hand, doctors are legally, ethically bound to obtain informed consent based on the correct information but on the other hand, they are contractually bound by the employer to not discuss insurance coverage of certain health. In the U.S., these are known as "gag" clauses – both lead to unpleasant consequences e.g. *do not discuss suggested treatments with members with insurance health plans before getting authorization*.

Tackling "gag" laws:

Due to aggressive legislative lobbying, there are some laws called "anti-gag laws". They have still not completely resolved the doctors' problems in this regard because many doctors are still "terminated without cause" from the panel of health organizations. This is harmful for the patients on many levels, e.g. by influencing doctors to divert patients away from acquiring cutting-edge, expensive or experimental treatments. However, it has damaged the doctor-patient relationship in the most grievous ways possible. The only legal remedy that can be offered is to make more vicious patient-friendly laws. Legally and ethically, the best advice is to **choose informed consent over legal liabilities with the health management organization**, i.e. make a few legal mistakes but always benefit the patient – discuss all possible treatment options with them. Dr. Yamaha in our scenario, did the right thing.

3. Defamation:

Let us see another scenario:

"Dr. Freeman is an orthopedic surgeon who has just completed his examination of the patient, Mr. Paul who has come to his orthopedic clinic with a complaint of severe lower back ache and bilateral sacroiliac joint dysfunction. Dr. Freeman records the history and completes the examination notes and according to him, Mr. Paul shows exaggerated pain behavior and uncertain signs on examination highlighting "malingering". He is being told by Mr. Paul that he needs a "certification" of disability as he is stuck in some litigation over his condition. When Dr. Freeman goes back to front office for dictating his notes to nurse and receptionist, Mr. Paul overhears him saying "Mr. Paul apparently has

no solid physical basis for his complaint. He is being very emotional seems to be prone to exaggeration. His illness seems psychological to me". Then he writes a prescription for depression. Mr. Paul's health plan refused to sponsor his treatment for depression and he filed a defamation suit against Dr. Freeman".

Defamation is a *"tort* **that develops a legal liability if one person attacks another's reputation"**

Its purpose is to safeguard one's reputation from damage that can occur by making false statements about the person to any third party/parties. *"Libels"* are written defamation while *"slander"* is verbal defamation. Doctors frequently get involved in circumstances where they can or do actually make harmful remarks about others' reputation. This law is somewhat more difficult to handle, than privacy breach laws. The defamation tort has an origin in English Law where "reputation" is seen as a fundamental component of a socioeconomic system.

Generally, courts all over the world, especially in U.S. are hesitant to question free speech unless any strong reason exists. Paradoxically, reputation of a person is extremely valuable to not only the person himself, but the society as well. Defamation is a tool to seek protection for a person's personal interests. Generally, these elements must be present in a defamation claim to hold weight:

   I. Presence of a defamatory statement:
      The statement against which a person is filing for defamation needs to be defamatory where the nature of defamation can be tested by asking certain questions: "as a result of hearing/reading this, would people think worse about the person (complainant)?"

   II. Defamatory statement must be false:
      In order for the statement be defamatory, it must not be true.

   III. A third party must be present to which the statement has to be communicated

   IV. The person making defamatory statements should know that the statement is false

   V. The person being filing for the defamation must be able to justify and prove that the defamation has directly brought harm to them e.g. an illness, psychological trauma, etc.

In several defamation cases, plaintiffs claim the doctors to be public figures and hence need bigger punishments. An example from the U.S. newspaper article half a century ago claimed that a doctor did not perform a procedure on a patient and was involved in "negligence", which led to complications, culminating in leg amputation of the patient. The law rejected the argument as the doctor was not a high-profile person in the medical community. In some other cases, the doctor who advertised himself as someone important into the public and enjoyed the limelight, was labelled by the court as a "public figure".

Other types of cases are where doctors disclose information about a patient to a third party. It may be done to let the third party know about the dangers the patient's disease condition might cause to the public. Such cases have also been unfruitful.

Age of technology has provided opportunities to allow claims of online defamation to happen. For example, for the republication of defamatory statements, an internet service provider was sued by a user. The court reasoned with the provider but also said that if the provider knew about the defamatory nature of statements, it would be rightly bound to stop it. More of such cases will follow if we keep on relying blindly on this form of communication.

Therefore, assessing the defamation scenario; it is evident that Dr. Freeman has disclosed some defamatory statements about Mr. Paul to the third party which can potentially harm his reputation. Two out of five elements of defamatory actions are present. Mr. Paul can also present some economic damages as proofs as his health plan was refusing his depression treatment based on Dr. Freeman's prescription and notes. The outcome? It will depend on whether Dr. Freeman was right or wrong about his assessment of Mr. Paul. Despite of the fact that Dr. Freeman's practice was not at all good, his statements could be defended falling within the *"professional judgement"* criteria.

It is therefore concluded that the patient's medical record is not place to judge, editorialize, blame or make off-hand remarks, and should be strictly discouraged.

Ethical issues in health communication

A practicing doctor has an undeniable responsibility to decide on patient care not in any one but several different type of surroundings. These decisions require selection of appropriate treatment and intervention options.

"Ethics" is *"an inherent, integral and inseparable part of practicing medicine"* as the physician has ethical obligations

  i. To benefit the patient

 ii. To not do harm or minimize harm

 iii. respect the social, cultural and religious values and preferences of the patient

Ethics is a broad term. It is a study of the nature of morals and making of specific moral choices.

"Normative ethics" can answer the question *"which general moral norms for the conduct guidance and evaluation should be accepted, and why?".* Some moral norms for "right" or "good" conduct are well-known and well-accepted to human kind as they are divided into many regions, religions, and identities: constitute *common morality* as shown in the figure.

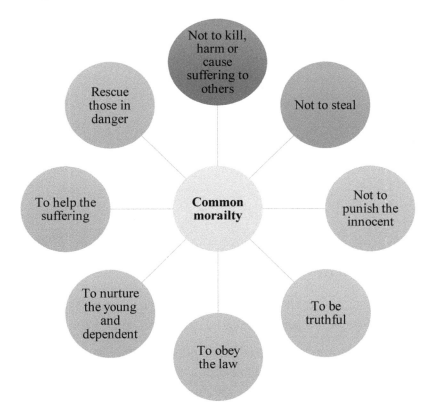

Attributes of common morality

Particular morality talks about the norms that connect different groups together due to their religion, profession, culture, and also deals with responsibilities, ideals, professional standards, etc. The best example is the doctor's **"accepted role"** or "supposed role" to provide efficient, reliable and trustworthy service to patients. To lessen the ambiguity of the term "accepted role", medical organization (local, state, national, international) have "codified" their acceptable standards for doctors' professional roles. However, **it may not always be**

possible for doctors to fulfil the moral responsibilities as the standards often prefer the professional duties over moral ones i.e. issues concerning patients and society.

Four principles of ethics in healthcare

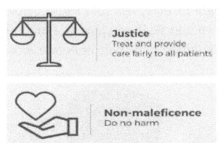

Justice
Treat and provide care fairly to all patients

Non-maleficence
Do no harm

Autonomy
Respect a person's freedom to choose what's right for them

Beneficence
All choices for a patient are made with the intent to do good

Bioethics and Clinical Ethics

Often, one of the most deplorable abuses of humans is in research, performing medical procedures without informed consent, concentration camps' experimentation in in World

War II, and salutary advancements in medicine and technology as well as societal changes. They all have led to rapid evolution of bioethics, from "professional code of conduct" to currently "clinical ethics, research ethics, organizational ethics, and public health ethics"

<u>The Fundamental Principles of Clinical Ethics</u>

The four fundamental principles of medical or bioethics and their implementation in clinical practice are mentioned below:

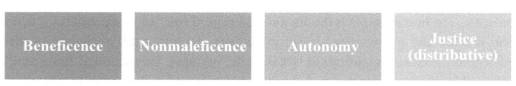

Four fundamental principles of medical ethics

Beneficence and nonmaleficence: *"to help and do no harm,"* can be traced down back to the time of *"Hippocrates of Kos"*, popularly known as *"Hippocrates"* (460 – 370 BC) *or Hippocrates II*, a Greek *physician* belonging to the classical period – one of the most brilliant figures in the history of medicine.

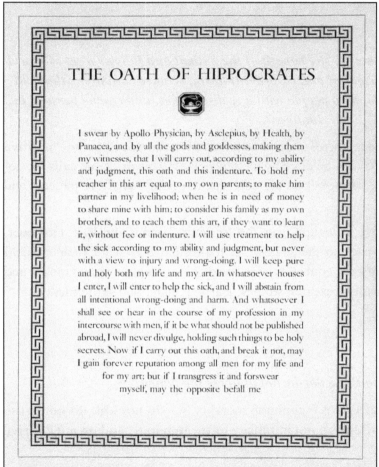

THE OATH OF HIPPOCRATES

I swear by Apollo Physician, by Asclepius, by Health, by Panacea, and by all the gods and goddesses, making them my witnesses, that I will carry out, according to my ability and judgment, this oath and this indenture. To hold my teacher in this art equal to my own parents; to make him partner in my livelihood; when he is in need of money to share mine with him; to consider his family as my own brothers, and to teach them this art, if they want to learn it, without fee or indenture. I will use treatment to help the sick according to my ability and judgment, but never with a view to injury and wrong-doing. I will keep pure and holy both my life and my art. In whatsoever houses I enter, I will enter to help the sick, and I will abstain from all intentional wrong-doing and harm. And whatsoever I shall see or hear in the course of my profession in my intercourse with men, if it be what should not be published abroad, I will never divulge, holding such things to be holy secrets. Now if I carry out this oath, and break it not, may I gain forever reputation among all men for my life and for my art; but if I transgress it and forswear myself, may the opposite befall me

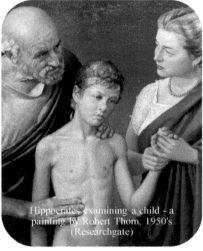

Hippocrates examining a child - a painting by Robert Thom, 1950's (Researchgate)

The latter two, autonomy and justice came into the light later. *Thomas Percival's* book on ethics *"Medical Ethics"* (1803) discussed the importance of patient's interest which according to him should be kept in his best interest and this should be the ultimate goal of patient care to be stressed upon. Autonomy and justice were not addressed. With time, both autonomy and justice bcame widely accepted as important principles of ethics.

In relatively **modern times,** *Thomas Beauchamp (1939—present)* and *James Childress (1940—present*), two American philosophers, who are best known for their work in medical ethics with their book *"Principles of Biomedical Ethics"* classically describes all these four principles and their implementation, also discussing alternative approaches.

1. Beneficence:

It can be defined as

"the obligation of the doctor to act for the benefit of the patient and follows a set of moral rules to guard and defend the right of others, prevent harm, remove conditions that will cause any damage to the people, help people with any disabilities, and rescue persons in danger".

It is distinct from nonmaleficence: here under "beneficence", the focus is on "positive requirements - the things which have to be done by the physician". This principle calls for not only preventing and avoiding the harm, but on the other hand, giving benefit to patients and promoting their welfare.

A doctor's beneficence must derive its weight from the "morality" and is altruistic. However, often, it can be viewed as a payback to the society for their contribution for their medical education (government's subsidized education for medical students), their ranks and privileges, and to patients, personally (research studies, learning, hands-on skill practice).

2. Nonmaleficence

Nonmaleficence is

"the obligation of a doctor not to harm the patient"

It seems to support various moral values ("common morality") – **do not kill, do not cause pain or suffering, do not cause offense, o not handicap or incapacitate, and do not deprive others of the goods of life.**

Nonmaleficence is the most "practical" implementation of for the doctor to compare benefits with burdens of all medical interventions and treatments, to get around the tough ones and to opt for the best action plan for the patient. The most practical and relevant example is the taking of "difficult end-of-life decisions" for patient care in such situations: whether to withhold or withdraw life-support and treatment, total parenteral nutrition and hydration; and in pain control in palliative care for advanced, inoperable cancers, etc.

A physician's commitment and intention to relieve the melancholy (e.g. pan refractory to conventional analgesics, or dyspnea) of a patient by using right drugs e.g. opioid analgesics overriding the predictable but unintended deleterious effects or consequences (***double-effect doctrine***).

3. Autonomy

Autonomy, as explained by philosophers ***Immanuel Kant (1724–1804) and John Stuart Mill (1806–1873)*** and well-renowned as an ethical principle, means that:

"all people have innate and unconditional worth, and therefore, should have the authority to make rational decisions and moral choices, and each should be permitted to exercise his or her measure for self-determination".

This ethical principle was reaffirmed by Justice Cardozo in the U.S. in 1914 with this succinct postulate: "Every human being of adult years and sound mind has a right to determine what shall be done with his own body"

Autonomy, like other principles, must weigh against other conflicting moral principles, and can be overrun, e.g. if the patient's action causes harm to another person(s) like patients with antisocial personality disorders. The principle does not apply to the people who do not possess the capability (competence) to act autonomously e.g. infants, children, and developmental/ mental/physical disorders leading to incompetence. There are certain procedures to assess incompetence. However, a distinct boundary exists between incapacity and incompetence. Incapacity is the inability to take healthcare decisions and is assessed by health professionals. Incompetence is determined by court of law0. Both of them are not practically valuable, as a doctor's assessment of a patient's incapacity based on physical or mental disorder has the same real-life repercussions as a lawful determination of incompetence.

4. Distributive justice

Justice is "fair, equitable, and appropriate treatment of persons"

There are several categories of justice but the one pertinent to clinical ethics is "distributive justice". Distributive justice can be explained as "equitable, just and appropriate availability of healthcare resources depending on justified norms that forms the basis of social cooperation". It can be accomplished by making sure that the three basic principles of distributive justice are followed. The healthcare resources are distributed to each person:

    i.   As an equal share

ii.   According to requirement

iii.   According to efforts

iv.   According to contribution

v.   According to merit

vi.   According to free-market exchanges

Being non-exclusive, each of these principles can be merged into each other for implementation, i.e. choosing, levelling and polishing them to form a synchronized and feasible to distribute medical resources with justice.

The practical examples include allotment of meagre resources (investigations, equipment, drugs, organ transplants), taking care of uninsured patients, and time allocation for OPD visits.

Beneficence, nonmaleficence	*Clinical assessment* Nature of illness (acute, chronic, reversible, terminal)? Goals of treatment? Treatment options and probability of success for each option? Adverse effects of treatment and does benefit outweigh harm? Effects of no medical/surgical treatment? If treated, plans for limiting treatment? Stopping treatment?
Respect for autonomy	*Patient rights and preferences* Information given to patient on benefits and risks of treatment? Patient understood the information and gave consent? Patent mentally competent? If competent, what are his/her preferences? If patient mentally incompetent, are patient's prior preferences known? If preferences unknown, who is the appropriate surrogate?
Beneficence, nonmaleficence, respect for autonomy	*Quality of life (QOL)* Expected QOL with and without treatment? Deficits – physical, mental, social – may have after treatment? Judging QOL of patient who cannot express himself/herself? Who is the judge? Recognition of possible physician bias in judging QOL? Rationale to forgo life-sustaining treatment(s)?
Distributive justice	*External forces and context* Conflicts of interests – does physician benefit financially, professionally by ordering tests, prescribing medications, seeking consultations? Research or educational considerations that affect clinical decisions, physician orders? Conflicts of interests based on religious beliefs? Legal issues? Conflicts of interests between organizations (clinics, hospitals), 3rd party payers? Public health and safety issues? Problems in allocation of scarce resources?

four principles of medical ethics - clinical examples

Effect of internet on the legal and ethical aspects of communication:

The world has become a "cyberspace" which is an environment where ever-changing, worldwide-linked, multilingual and multicultural information exists. It challenges and dodges all the traditional limitations of the humankind, be it borders, ethical and cultural standards, laws, rules and regulations. Following this in to the health sector, drug-relations have been has jeopardized due to drugs being sold and purchased all over the internet in the name of "self-care". Unlimited and unrestricted access is being provided to the masses regarding the information and health products in the name of "alternative medicines". All this has destabilized the age-old, classic 'doctor-patient relationship".

Internet gives unfathomable power to the people to share any kind of healthcare information with patients, other healthcare professionals, their families, primary caregivers, educators, research students, insurers, policymakers, legislators and regulators. And they do so with immaculate timeliness, depth, accuracy and diversity. These qualities make the internet a rich, dense marketplace of creativity and ideas.

Due to a decentralization provided by the internet, its global web reach, unlimited access to publication tools, possibility of responding immediately and facilitation of interchange, renders it an exceptional capability to spread potential "misinformation", hidden bias, unethical usage, secret dealings, fraudulent activities, and last but not the least, illegal escape from taxes and regulations.

Digging deeper, it has been found out that the efforts to control unethical practices in healthcare over the internet are inadequate, at both national and international levels. Special emphasis should be laid on "jurisdiction" – a problem that needs an urgent solution. An internationally accepted policy framework should be developed that lays out the basic rights and responsibilities of users as well as providers. Critical topics to be covered are "freedom of expression and information access" and "protection of privacy and data security of the user". To deal with cyberspace's legal and ethical problems in health and healthcare, important steps need to be taken. Experts of civil and criminal law, bioethics, medical ethics, medical computing, legal medicine and computing ethics must be involved.

Patient Privacy:

Healthcare information is a matter of great sensitive nature. Knowing this fact, health professionals and health-related organizations should pay special attention to reliability of patient's medical records and any issues with patient's integrity, security, privacy, and confidentiality must be effectively addressed.

There are two factors make this matter extremely important: inherently-sensitive patient data and the heavy use of internet for processing of healthcare information. Off-site processing and data storage of electronic health records by services providers, makes it particularly unsafe.

Safeguarding the safety and integrity of patient data and organization's health network should be the top priority. In fact, the use of internet for health data management systems should fulfil several prerequisites or guarantees: privacy and confidentiality of every patient's health information, content quality, consumer protection and industry's commercial interests online, will be guarded from unethical practices.

There are many aspects and issues pertaining to patient's privacy which has unwaveringly been one of the top concerns of users. "Health data banks" have given rise to user's fears of breach in privacy, right of access and use of personal data. Some countries have enacted privacy laws which allows individuals to know which information is being stored, who can access it and how erroneous information. that information, and mechanism of correction of erroneous information - authenticity, reliability, and accuracy. There are more than 20000 websites related to health and most of them are profit-driven which can and do promote unproven, dangerous products and treatments. Others may not intend to harm but contain misleading and wrong information. It is extremely difficult to label websites as credible or not credible, motives good or find out about their sponsorship.

Somewhere in the center of this all, internet-friendly patients bombard freely available or "free-for-all," doctors during consultation with a plethora of information learnt over the internet. They sometimes bring along downloaded information and are interested in discussing their *"self-diagnosed"* conditions and recommendations for alternative treatments.

Although electronic transactions do not address all legal and regulatory problems, but they address plenty, nevertheless. In marketing, promotion and sale of medical products online, vigilance is required for the maintenance of legal and ethical standards. Some of these standards include:

- Approval of health products (herbal, nutrient, etc.), health devices, and pharmaceutical drugs by the relevant regulatory authorities of the buyer's region or country
- Determination of the place of transaction (buyer's or seller's jurisdiction)
- Determination of the court of law which will settle disputes if arises.

Ethical and legal aspects in telemedicine:

Everyone agrees to having the ethical and legal regulations standardized and introduction of "seal of approval" but their implementation is still a hazy area, especially across the borders where jurisdiction is not addressed by laws or regulations. A number of international organizations have been active in this regard: Health on the Net Foundation, Internet Healthcare Coalition American Medical Association, and European medical societies.

We know that data security, privacy, and confidentiality are concerning matters in clinical applications which are telecommunication-based. However, they also raise squabble in terms of professional behavior, accountability, technical standards, licensure, and reimbursement. Some other issues which can arise are model of care, liability, malpractice and negligence as telemedicine involves several health providers who are geographically far away and come under diverse ethical practices and legal systems.

The society and public authorities should encourage *"public good"* to be made universally available for fulfilling social, educational and cultural needs. The challenge is to define concepts such as "universal access" and "public domain", implement and promote them for public welfare. However, private initiatives must also be encouraged to protecting personal rights of people, their dignity, intellectual property rights, fair usage, and rights to economic claims.

Usually local standards are used as parameters to evaluate health practice as well as litigation. Remote conduction of medical consultation and interventions bring its own legal and ethical problem in telecare patient-doctor relationship. Unfortunately, no guidelines exist now but they are being developed several professional, technical and trade organizations, internationally.

Licensing and regulation of healthcare workers is being done in many countries via e-commerce. Validation of their practicing licenses, alternative/non-certified health practice, fraudulent practice and deceitful are regulatory and quality assurance problems that need to be assessed.

Healthcare organizations are fully responsible for and must ensure complete safety of patient security, privacy, and confidentiality, even in the face of the growing challenges. Conflicts based on data sharing, security and confidentiality must be resolved while procuring the health system after implementation. security features must be incorporated into the management systems. It is still unfortunate that there are no written rules and regulations for authorization of accessing client information e.g. organization policy on sensitive information disclosure or disciplinary actions for violation.

Countries belonging to the developing part of the world are particularly and significantly afflicted with this rapid and uncontrollable explosion of communication via IT. The government, non-government, private, advocacy firms, healthcare industry and general users have raised in some questions about the impact of this rapid shift to technology.

The most problematic aspect is lack of trust over the reliability of healthcare information, innovative health practice, advertising and marketing processes, content validity and privacy, over internet. Not much has been done to address this, hence, ethical and legal issues still exist.

The United Nations (especially UNESCO), the World Health Organization (WHO), the International Telecommunications Union (ITU), the World Trade Organization (WTO), regional trade blocks of European Union, NAFTA, MERCOSUR, and World Bank and Inter-American Development Bank have sponsored to initiate the development of regulations for practicing telemedicine.

Sources:

1. Rodrigues R. Ethical and legal issues in interactive health communications: a call for international cooperation. J Med Internet Res. 2000 Jan-Mar;2(1):E8. doi: 10.2196/jmir.2.1.e8. PMID: 11720927; PMCID: PMC1761840
2. Shomaker, T; Ashburn, MA. The Legal Implications of Healthcare Communications: What Every Pain Physician Needs to Know. Pain Medicine. 1(1):89–96
3. Varkey B: Principles of Clinical Ethics and Their Application to Practice. Med Princ Pract 2021;30:17-28. doi: 10.1159/000509119

PRESENTATION SKILLS IN HEALTHCARE

Chapter 6

Delivering a great presentation in healthcare - Tips and Tricks

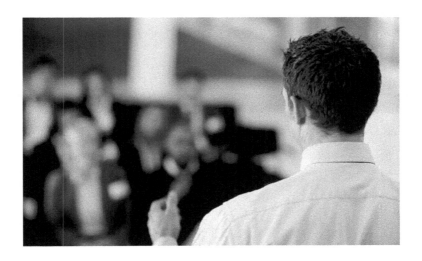

Presenting in the modern era:

This is an era of technology, and the modern man has been advancements in almost all fields of medicine and modalities of management: lab investigations, other diagnostic modalities, drugs, interventions, research, medical education, etc. In the same way, delivering presentations in healthcare has also evolved over time and has become dependent on technology now. Presentation, as name suggests, is an art of presenting the information to an audience. The key, however, is doing it efficiently, confidently, fluently and artfully. There are many purposes to be achieved through presentations in healthcare.

The methods for presentations have changed over time. From verbal presentation to charts to black board to white board to transparencies to multimedia and now interactive real-time presentations. Even if we talk about PowerPoint presentations, Microsoft has been updating and empowering it for many years, with innovative and unique features, so as to enable it to become more user-friendly, efficient and visually appealing with stunning graphics.

Let us introduce ourselves to Microsoft PowerPoint.

Introduction to Microsoft PowerPoint – one of the most important tools in Microsoft Office

Microsoft PowerPoint is a presentation software that was created by **Robert Gaskins** and **Dennis Austin** at a software startup in Silicon Valley named **Forethought, Inc.** It was released on April 20, 1987. PowerPoint, later, became a component of the Microsoft Office suite, first offered in 1990 for Windows, which bundled several Microsoft apps. Beginning with PowerPoint 4.0 in 1994, PowerPoint was incorporated into Microsoft Office development, and adopted shared common components and a converged user interface.

Operation - Key features:

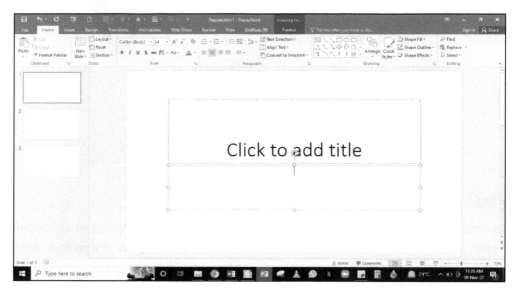

Microsoft PowerPoint user interface for a blank presentation

Contemporarily, MS PowerPoint is used to create a *"file"* (blank presentation, based on a template, etc.), also known as *"presentation"* or *"deck"*, that contains a series of pages called *"slides"*. They usually have a consistent style (created from designs known as *template masters*), and contain information either imported from other applications or created exclusively in PowerPoint: *text, bullet lists, images, drawn shapes, audio clips, tables, charts, graphs, text-to-speech option, video clips, animations of elements, and animated transitions between slides*, plus *attached notes* for each slide.

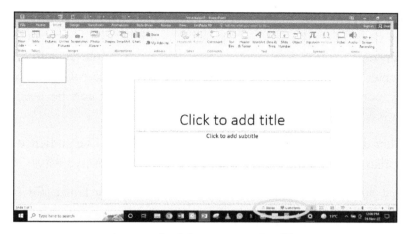

insert tab of the presentation file

After a file is created, it is very easy and a typical operation to present it as a **"slide show"** or **"presentation mode"** using a portable computer. The presentation file is either stored on the computer, available from a network or stored in USB on a computer. One can also switch to **"projection mode"** from the **"settings"** option in control panel. There are many modes of projection: **PC screen only, duplicate view, extended view and second screen only**. To see the presentation on both the projection screen and the computer/laptop, duplicate view is chosen.

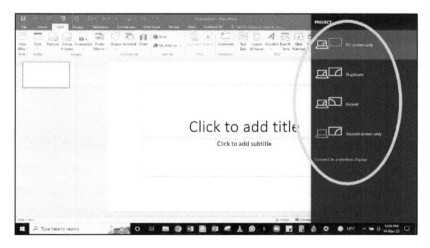

Modes of projection

The **computer's or laptop's screen** shows a **"presenter view"** with current slide, next slide, speaker's notes for the current slide, and information like time since the start of slide show. The video is sent from the computer to one or more external **digital projectors** or **monitors,**

showing only the current slide to the audience (notes are also not visible to the audience), with the speaker controlling the sequencing at the computer. A smartphone remote-control built in to PowerPoint for **iOS** (optionally controlled from Apple Watch) and for **Android** allows the presenter to control the show from elsewhere in the room. Also there are slide changers simply connected via USB into the computers and can be used to control the sequence from anywhere in the room (within a range).

Additionally, other than a computer slide shown projected to a live audience by the speaker, PowerPoint can also be used to present in numerous other impressive ways:

- Displayed on the screen of the presentation computer or tablet (for limited audience e.g. small group discussions)
- Printed for distribution as supportive paper documents (in many printable formats)
- Shared and distributed as files for private viewing, even on computers that don't have PowerPoint
- Shared on freelancing websites like Freelancer, Fiverr, Upwork, Slideshare, etc.
- Shared on social media platforms like Facebook or Twitter
- Set up as a self-running unattended display
- Shared in a webpage or blog
- Recorded as video/audio to be distributed as for any other video
- Broadcasted live presentation over the web
- Packaged for distribution on CD or a network as linked and embedded data

There are many *tips and tricks* which can be taught and learned when it comes to delivering excellent Microsoft presentation

Presenting with Microsoft PowerPoint – When and Where?

Presentations using Microsoft PowerPoint are not only used to inform or educate people, but also to train and convince different internal and external audiences. Clinical practice includes some easy and some difficult explanations, therefore, the healthcare presentations are for a very wide audience. One can create a healthcare presentation for both children and scientists.

Words and correctly used animations have a great power. Most complex concepts can be explained to audience (or students) e.g. movement of a white blood cell from circulation to the site of inflammation. Here is a list of occasions and situations where presentations are essential in healthcare.

i. Ward meetings

ii. Journal clubs

iii. Mortality meetings

iv. Teaching in medical schools (physical as well as online)

- Large group interactive sessions

- Small group interactive sessions

v. To present research findings

vi. Webinars

vii. Medical conferences

viii. Demonstrating a new equipment or medical services presentation

ix. Delivering medical case presentations (departmental, interdepartmental, clinic-pathological conferences as a routine academic activity in teaching hospitals)

x. Workshops

xi. Medical training

xii. Seminars

xiii. Medical networking

xiv. Medical investment pitch

xv. Medical TED talk

xvi. Medical invention demonstration.

There are numerous other occasions where medical or healthcare presentations can be utilized. In short, anytime you talk about healthcare problems or new information, you need a medical presentation.

Presentation in healthcare

Presenting medical topics is often believed to be "difficult", more so without Microsoft PowerPoint. So, PowerPoint presentations must be used smartly and wisely to make the speech and content easier to understand. For explaining simpler concepts, presentation can be a life-saver if approached in a meaningful way.

How to make your next PowerPoint (PPT) presentation a success: tips and tricks

The presentation goals can be reached with proper planning, preparation, smart work and confidence.

Quick Steps:

Step 1: Rely on the visuals

- Look for the visuals that can accompany and complement your text
- PowerPoint was originally created for animation, but a lot of people use slides incorrectly and make paragraphs filled with scientific information.
- It has been observed that humans grasp visual information 60,000 times more rapidly than pure and simply written text
- So, whenever technical presentation is need to be presented, the audience would always want and prefer relevant visual aids to reinforce their understanding.
- For example: do not just name types of bone fractures or blood cells, instead, show them!

Step 2: Always present clean and clear images by cropping and enlarge them

- An extension of the first step: it is recommend using one picture per ed to use one slide per slide; Enlarging would help if it contains small elements
- For example, a cataract needs to be shown: increase the image size for all people to see clearly
- f you have to, always sacrifice the text for a clear, big, high-quality picture

Step 3: Use charts to visualize numbers

- Avoid using numeorus bullet points and endless lists on slides
- Decide how many numbers or statistics are to be added as separate slides
- Do not intermingle pictures with charts/graphs.
- Make them simple but clear.
- it is better to use contrasting backgrounds and comment on every picture (art)
- Bullet points are good in making some space and differentiation in an otherwise long, monotonous text

Step 4: Give professional look to your graphics

- Search online for templates and tutorials for medical presentation to improve PowerPoint presentation
- There will be expectations if you need to present in front of other professionals
- Use high-resolution HD images, position every element on the slide accordingly
- Sizes of the arrow and lines, spacing should be uniform - match them
- Remove all the foreign, irrelevant elements that pollute the animation.

Eight simple tips to improve healthcare presentation

Although, these eight simple tips and tricks to make better healthcare PowerPoint presentations are very easy to implement, but they will have a significant impact on the quality of medical slides, as well as boost your confidence.

1. Thinking "Non-Linear":

While showing and explaining some definitions, do not present them in a boring and linear way. It will easily lead to the "disengagement" of the audience from the slide or later, presentation. Instead, an animated explanation can be created with arrows: and the important word can be made "big and prominent" in the middle of the slide. The definition should be 'drawn' around it. After all if you have PowerPoint, why use only the words?

2. Using simple animated visuals to make the audience grasp concepts

For example, you have to explain how some drug molecules cross the cell membranes, a plethora of hard-to-understand, monotonous text does not attract anyone among the audience. For better people engagement, one can draw how charged drug molecules move forward and back. Besides, the point is that the visual memory is better than verbal memory and in this way, they will grasp it better through "visualization". Thus, the information sticks to the audience's brains and keeps their attention tightly clutched till the presentation ends.

3. Labelling your images right

Images are a very important and game-changing part of any medical presentation, provided they are used wisely. Unfortunately, some presenters don't use them smartly and create eye hops. It can be explained by the number of things eyes have to be laid on in a single slide to make sense of the information and gather it. Always *"think about the audience"* when making a presentation. And try to see from their eyes, to imagine how their eyes will drift through the slide. The presenter should make their way as easy as possible. For example, when you label parts of an esophagus, it will not be wise to create a 1-5 list next to the picture. It can make people weary, having to move their eyes from the picture to the list and back again to the picture. It is better to label parts with names immediately. The presenter should let the audience perceive the information step-wise.

4. Use tables for comparison

We know, bullet points are good to save space on a sliced as it is limited. So, it looks better if custom animations are applied using the bullet points, save space and still present in a linear way. In accordance with this save-saving and presenting with simplicity principle, it is advised that a "table" should be used instead of bullet points. It will also be a better choice if one has to compare two items with a column that explains the characteristics you oppose. It allows the audience to follow the presenter's thoughts to different levels. Let the people understand and connect. If they don't connect, they get distracted faster and any presenter should not let that happen

5. Pay attention to the clarity of information

It should be ensured that the images that have been placed on the slide are matching with the main headlines or the text on the slide. Sometimes, it happens that people put too much information in one slide i.e. both images and lots of text, because they fear making "too many slides". And they have no idea about or try to ignore that the audience in the back seats cannot see anything.

6. Use charts for presenting numbers

Let us take an example where some information regarding the etiological factors of a disease is to be presented. Instead of quoting percentage, show them!! Visual information is perceived better than plain text. So, to understand and remember the information regarding numbers and percentages, charts can be used to share percentages of each factor. Remember, the PowerPoint was initially created for animations, so always look for strategies to avoid many words and lots of plain text and numbers.

7. Lead with appropriate visuals

If the presentation is being delivered to general audience only for information purpose or any other nonacademic purpose, it is not advisable to display the photos of bad wounds, severely disfiguring skin or organ diseases, or other health problems. It may cause aversion in some people because the pictures aren't really pleasing to the sight and don't serve any purpose. Instead, "drawn pictures" can be used, e.g. do not show classification on real skin but on cross-section (like in medicine books).

8. Avoid Using Photos as Slide Backgrounds

Oddly though, many medical presenters use pictures as background for some reason. It is however, not recommended and not advisable: it is supposed to be extremely hard for the audience to differentiate the text from the image (or words in the image) – it all seems to be quite clogged up. Background photos do not bring much importance. Simplicity is always the best policy. So, the simpler, the better.

Presenting in healthcare – a conclusion:

Eye-catching animations always add an element of attraction to any medical presentation, even if one has doubts, it has surely never spoiled anyone's presentation. By adding subtle, suitable colors and pictures for a neat look, the expertise can be demonstrated and speech can be supported. In this way, the presenter will not get lost even if any interruption occurs. Some complex topics are explained better if the visuals are attractive most all people understand information accompanied by visuals better than words alone. Therefore, this preference needs to be applied on any kind of audience, of any size, age, and gender

Sources:

1. https://slidepeak.com/blog/tips-for-engaging-medical-presentation
2. https://en.wikipedia.org/wiki/Microsoft_PowerPoint
3. https://en.wikipedia.org/wiki/Adult_Learning
4. "How to run seminars and workshops: presentation skills for consultants, trainers, and teachers" by Robert L. Jolles

Chapter 7

Preparations before your presentation

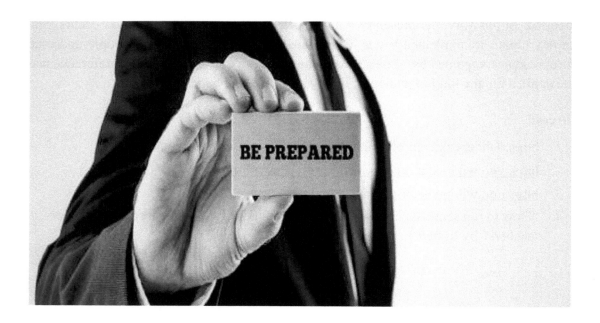

Before a presentation

What is a presentation? *It is more than just a mere opportunity to introduce an idea*. Rather, it *is introduction, discussion and explanation of one's viewpoints, convictions and opinion*. It is a means to substantiate and demonstrate the hard work and research a person has invested into. And when it comes to preparing for a presentation, let it be any presentation, one needs to remember that the way the presentation will be delivered is of prime important (perhaps even more so) than the actual content of the presentation.

Preparing to present the information needs many important things to be kept in mind. As discussed above, the focus should be on the "way" of presentation than on the content itself. The "art" of presentation, like all the other arts is based on "skill", one might as well call it a "performing art". It needs a high level of talent, confidence, practice, charisma, knowledge, eloquence, fluency, power of persuasion, and intelligence.

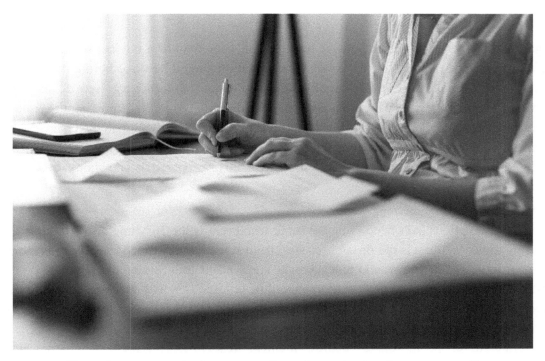

Yes, what you say isn't necessarily as important as how you say it.

How to get ready for a presentation?

Whenever you will think back to the last good presentation you attended, the one that had you gripped for days and you kept thinking about it for many days afterwards - you should ask yourselves: what made it so persuasive? What made it so compelling? How and why did it motivate you? Why did inspire you?

This is mainly because the speaker or presenter "engaged" you. That was no luck or chance. This was no coincidence. He must have work hard for it to happen. Practice makes a man perfect.

So, it is now known by a lot of people that a ton of hard work and preparation goes on behind the scenes of an excellent, memorable presentation. What many people may not realize is that this preparation stage goes even further, beyond jotting down some notes and practicing in front of a mirror.

A stellar presentation takes a lot of time, stamina, effort, energy and last but not the least, a lot of practice. Here are the key things that must be done before any presentation:

1. Doing the research:

Regardless of the fact whether you are an expert in your field or a novice, some new things are always there to be learnt. A thorough investigation should be done before plotting your presentation, to make sure if there is anything new about that topic: e.g. new developments relevant to your subject or your audience. Another important thing is "knowing the content". Make sure your knowledge about your material is excellent. It will abolish the chances of any uncertainly and the dreaded gestures like "umnms" and "uhhhs" that are not liked by anyone. These gestures show that you're not as knowledgeable or prepared as you should be.

2. Knowing your audience

No two presentations ever need to be the same whether it is the 20th time one is talking about the same topic. While it is not possible to start from scratch every time you have to present on the same topic again, you should at least make some effort into finding out who will be there sitting in the audience. The presentation should be tailored in a way that will appeal to them. Therefore, every presenter should focus the most on the fact that the information about to be shared is according to what the audience can comprehend. For example, are there undergraduate or postgraduate medics, medical academics, researchers, pharmaceutical representatives, trainees, registrars, consultants, administrators, nurses, receptionists, patients, their families or community. Everyone has a different level of understanding for any given topic. So the information-sharing needs to be done in a way that the audience would understand it.

3. Crafting your notes

A good rule of thumb for any presentation is: If you cannot present without writing it down, you probably can't do it. You don't need to write a speech. Instead, craft important notes to rehearse your speaking points. Take quick glances at them from time to time to keep yourself on track. Revise and practice your notes every day until you don't need to look at them anymore (but it is advisable to take the notes with you anyway, the pressure of presenting can make people forgetful in front of a crowd.

4. Practicing your delivery

As mentioned above, notes will help you in preparing the content you are going to present but whatever you will "say" will not guarantee audience engagement. So what you can do is grab a camera, or cell phone and get in front of it, record yourself delivering your presentation and be your own critic. Give yourself an honest critique. This will make you realize about your shortcomings in the presentation style. Ask yourself questions: do you use body language effectively? Do you stroll around or remain static to the podium? Do you interact enough with the crowd? Is your posture appropriate? If you are not able to do a critical analysis of yourself, nominate a friend to take a look and help you point out the areas for improvement. Then practice, practice and keep on practicing.

5. Dress for success

Or you can say *"dress to impress"*. As I have mentioned before, nothing about the presentation is "co-incidental" and every bit of a great presentation is "intentional", including the dressing choice of the speaker. For example, a politician is speaking to blue collar workers (trying to appeal to them) and when you see them the next time, notice what color they will be wearing? A shirt with a blue collar and sleeves rolled up. The attire of the presenter must match or at least relate with the attire of the majority of the audience. Delivering a speech in a tuxedo or at ground-breaking ceremony of a developmental project just does not make sense.

6. Getting a good night's sleep

Make sure you look fresh, alert and sharp. This will only happen when you will take ample rest at night before a presentation. A slow, drowsy mind is a forgetful mind. And the tired eyes will not do you any good.

7. Preparing your space

Always reach the venue of presentation with enough time in your hands, ahead of your presentation, in order to properly prepare the space that will be used be used. Ensure that your slides are in order and that the equipment (if you are using), is functioning properly to avoid unnecessary delays, interruptions and embarrassing hiccups during your presentation. Play your videos, animations to check if they are playing fine. The speaking notes should be in a logical and accessible spot and get yourself a glass of water to avoid your throat from drying. Spend a few quiet minutes mentally preparing.

8. Being the speaker who inspires you

Public speaking or "oration" is a God-gifted talent and not everyone is a good speaker. The presenters can take cues and ideas form other professional speakers for their own presentation. While leaning anything in any field of life, it is always better to learn from the best. Everyone has heard or watched a speaker who has inspired them. You can also think back to the speeches you have heard or the people who have attracted you to their style of presenting. Strive and try to connect with your audience the same way that they make that same connection with your audience. Preparation is key. No presentation becomes an overnight success without preparation. So, invest some time into your presentation and audience.

9. Giving outline to your presentation

Write a valid sequence of the contents of your presentation to highlight them at the start of your presentation to catch the attention of the audience and give them a chance to try to understand the concept you will build later.

10. Timely practice of the presentation, comfortably ahead of time:

"Practice makes a man perfect", we have all heard that. The more the presenter practices, the more perfectly the presentation will be delivered. It is also advisable to practice in front of either a mirror or in front of a peer, friend, or colleague to boost confidence.

11. Reading and revising your presentation:

Reading the content of the presentation again and again will only tighten the grip of the presenter on the difficult concepts or sentences. Revising will not only boost the confidence, but will develop fluency and eloquence to his style of presentation.

12. Arriving in time for presentation:

Arriving well in time or even early before the start of the presentation gives the presenters the opportunity to settle themselves. It is good to start presentation in a relaxed and calculated, almost in a methodical kind of a way rather than appearing rushed, flustered, late or anxious.

13. Practicing hand gestures:

Before the presentation, the presenter should practice the hand gestures he will use during the session. Use of too much hand gestures is neither recommended nor looks nice. Hand gestures distract the audience. Gestures signify what is known as the "body language" and this is something really important to master during any presentation or even a routine professional communication.

14. Taking some deep breaths:

Anyone can feel anxious and flustered before the start of their presentation. Taking deep breaths is a way to fight off that nervousness, and makes the presenter relaxed.

Your presentation method

The presentation method is how you deliver a presentation.

It is just as important as preparing and organizing the material before your presentation. How the message is delivered is a vital component than the message itself. The goal should be to engage your audience and persuade them to give attention, listen and act on what you're saying. For this very reason, you need to spend some time into searching for and implementing the best presentation method.

Why presentation methods matter?

Connecting with audience is very important. We talk a lot about it because there is a very small value in presenting if the audience is not paying attention to what you're saying. When a presenter connects with the audience, he governs and commands their attention. They have no option but to listen to you. It is because you have "triggered" something in them that compels them to want to hear what you have to say. Most of the times, whatever clutches their attention is not just your words but how you speak them.

Presentation methods:

What exactly is meant by a "presentation method"? Well, let us consider the presentations you have delivered or those which you have attended. Remember that even a healthcare presentation has a lot of different shapes and sizes: variable topics, contexts, purposes and requirements, according to the department – however, coming back to the basics, any transfer of information between two or more people is a "presentation". And certainly, presentation methods vary according to their purposes. A healthcare presentation in workshops and seminars are different as compared to an academic presentation delivered by an academic in a medical school. A clinical fellow will present in a different way as compared to a pharmaceutical representative marketing his product.

Choosing a presentation method:

Think Ahead

Let us assume that you have already made some progress with the preparation of your presentation. The presentation content has been organized and plotted, the next step is to consider the way of delivering it. You may want to make a good impression by showing some videos in the beginning but before wowing your audience, wait a minute: does this venue or system have the audio equipment for playing the video sound?

So, as you start to map out your presentation method, you'll need to pay attention to the following factors:

a) The occasion

Every presentation has a unique purpose. No matter if it is being delivered on the same topic for a hundredth time, remind yourself that while the content may be the same for more than one situation, the occasion directs the presentation method. Match your presentation method according to the occasion.

b) The Audience

Once again, no matter how many times the same content has been presented on the same topic, the presentation needs to be tailored with respect to the audience of the day. If you are familiar with the people in the group and their knowledge on the subject, it will be helpful. Any formal event may have audience with little knowledge of the topic may need slides. However, a small and informal group who already are familiar with the topic or has an extensive knowledge of the subject, may just need infographics.

c) Venue of presenting

The importance of preparing your method according to venue can be imagined by assuming that you have applied for a job as a medical academician. You are required to present before a panel so that they can check your presentation skills. You thought that the presentation will be presented in a small 12 by 12 office in front of the official selection board. However, when you reach the venue, you find out that the venue is pretty big i.e. a lecture hall. The method for delivery which you will choose will be relative to the venue in which you will be presenting. Range of view, acoustics, and even the ambiance is different. If you can find out ahead of the time where exactly you'll be presenting, you can plan accordingly.

d) Availability of sound equipment

Any good presenter always makes sure that he tests his equipment before officially starting the presentation. This should be done before the time. Whether if it is just a collar microphone you need or more sophisticated equipment, ensure that you have the accurate knowledge about what equipment will be available to you before choosing your presentation method and how to operate it.

e) Availability of visual aids

Now, all over the world, most conference rooms are equipped with audio-video equipment, but it will not hurt to do a last-minute check on that before putting together a presentation that is dependent on PowerPoint slides

f) Preparation according to the level of interaction during the presentation

If the presentation is expected to be interactive and audience may be involved through participation, the presentation method needs to be selected accordingly. If you will be needing the audience members to be invited and share their experiences or participate in role-playing scenarios, you may need to walk around and reach into the audience. If it is not possible, at least ensure that you do not stick to only the stage the entire time. It is advisable to consider the methodology through which you will be interacting with your audience before choosing a presentation method.

g) Leave Nothing to Chance

A presentation needs to be carefully planned and prepared in order to be effective and successful (based on the venue, the type of audience and your objectives). Your goal should be to deliver a presentation that will captivate the audience and leave a durable impression on them. So, be strategic while choosing a presentation method and do some research before you choose.

Summarizing, there are many different methods to choose for deliver a memorable presentation. The key is in the preparing, approaching proactively regarding the methods and style of delivery and foreseeing the possible glitches.

Before preparing a presentation, it is important to assess yourself if you have a fear of speaking in public.

Fear of public speaking

People talk about "fear of public speaking" a lot, and there is a valid reason for that. A great percentage of people we interact and work with have *"glossophobia"* – *"fear of public speaking"*.

People employed in healthcare are considered to be very confident, outspoken and fluent in conversation, as they speak with a lot of people throughout the day. If we talk about doctors only, they deal with different kinds of population groups: administrative staff, healthcare staff, their health team members, medical students, their trainees, their nursing staff, their own family members and their patients. But are all doctors good public speakers as well? Are all doctors confident enough and never fear speaking in public? No.

It will not be wrong to say that a large and significant proportion of world's population admits to being afraid of public speaking. Can this be true? Can this many people really be paralyzed with fear of talking to other people? Something so ordinary? Then what to believe when there are a lot of teachers, speakers, actors, singers and politicians out there? Hard to believe but they must only make up the remaining little proportion of population, collectively.

The truth: most of the people who assume they fear speaking in public, really don't fear it all they are afraid because they suffer from *"stage fright"*.

Stage Fright: What is it?

"Stage fright" or "performance anxiety" is

"when a person feels afraid of performing in some way after he is asked to do so"

And the most common **"performance"** that sparks this fear of claiming the stage is **"public speaking"**. Paradoxically, some people do exist who perform or speak publically all the time but also suffer from stage fright? Many actors, public speakers and actors have confessed that they have had stage fright all their lives.

But suffering from stage fright doesn't strictly mean that one cannot speak publically. It's the "anticipation" of the event or performance, not the "act or speech" itself, that handicaps people with an overwhelming fear.

- **Separate your fear**

  You are a doctor who is very confident in your day-to-day communications but you feel public speaking triggers your stage fright, then can these two situations be disintegrated so you can go on to deliver a presentation confidently. The answer is a BIG yes.

- **Accept the fear**

  One step at a time. Start by recognizing the problem. Once you realize that your fear is directly-linked to presentation delivery (not the presentation itself), accept it as a part of the process. Don't tell yourself that you are not nervous - it won't work. If you admit and expect to be nervous, only then you can – put in the maximum effort and prepare your presentation and choose an appropriate delivery method. But that does not mean that you begin by letting your audience know that you are nervous (audience doesn't know, most of the times, if you don't tell them)

- **Put your adrenalin rush to work**

  It is quite natural to have your heart pound at the thought of having to stand up and start talking in public. That is cause by the fight-or-flight response (adrenaline rush) due to the activation of the sympathetic nervous system. It is an incredible thing to allow us to cope with the stress. Think: it's a jolt of energy. It can be used to cripple you or to inject energy into your presentation. I suggest the latter.

- **Rationalize the situation**

  Fear is also an innate emotion and response of the body's natural fight-or-flight (sympathetic) system to any stress or threat. When someone is in any dangerous situation, adrenaline is responsible for providing you the energy to run away or fight for survival or safety. So, even if you are stammering and fumbling the presentation, it will still be ok. It will pass.

- **Go Easy on Yourself**

  You prepare your presentation by investing time on it, so that you do it well. Everyone goes into a presentation with the intention of doing it well. No one wants to fumble through their notes and bore their audience. But here's the thing: nor every outcome can be anticipated, nor can you control all the things during your presentation. Practicing with PowerPoint to put slides are in order and equipment is operating is advisable, but there still may be things that can happen which will be out of your control. You cannot expect your presentation to be perfect, because it will cause disappointment: do not aim for perfection, aim for excellence.

- **Do It Often**

  Try to avail every opportunity to practice pubic speaking, even if it's a brief introduction of you and your work/profession. If you will do it more and more, and allow yourself to be exposed to it often, even if you will not overcome it, the fear will still get mitigated.

Do not let stage fright stop you from gaining your potential of becoming a powerful public speaker, all the lost opportunities will follow. Embrace the fears so you can use your fears to your advantage.

Making a presentation – rules for constructing an excellent PowerPoint presentation

To deliver an effective presentation, you need to take control of the *three main elements* of the event:

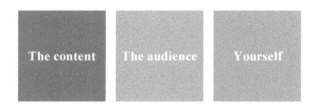

The skill of persuasion will be needed, no matter what the topic of your presentation is. You will need to:

   i. *Work out your big ideas: your content, your message*

  ii. *Validate your message using SPQR technique (situation–problem–question–response)*

 iii. *Arrange your ideas in a coherent fashion*

 iv. *Express your ideas vividly*

  v. *Remember your ideas, message and purpose*

 vi. *Deliver well*

Making a Presentation

Convert the nervous energy inside you into the performance itself. Preparing well is the key and the presentation will be brought to life. You can prepare in three core areas mentioned above:

1. **The material**
2. **The audience**
3. **Yourself**

In each case, **preparation** means ***taking control of your content and yourself***. Remove the elements of uncertainty in these two areas and you will be ready to encounter what cannot be controlled: ***the relationship between you and your audience.***

<u>Constructing PowerPoint slides - avoiding the pitfalls of bad slides</u>

Although there are many important things to keep in mind while delivering an excellent presentation, whether a clinical or a purely academic one, the most important of them all is making clear and attractive PowerPoint slides. No matter how clear in speech or confident the presenter is, poorly constructed slides can be regarded as the biggest pitfall in the art of presentations.

Imagine that you have to advise a new medical/dental lecturer on things to do and things not to do in making good PowerPoint slides (or you can imagine that you are the lecturer yourself!!!!).

- **You will need to make two lists (brainstorm some ideas)**
- **Group your ideas under similar headings (analyze the information you need to share)**
- **Share your ideas: in their turn, two new points per group.**

In this section, we will discuss the following aspects of slide construction:

1. *Outline*
2. *Slide Structure*
3. *Fonts*
4. *Color*
5. *Background*
6. *Graphs*
7. *Copyrighting*
8. *Spelling and Grammar*
9. *Conclusions*
10. *Questions*

Section of the presentation	Description	Examples
Outline	The topic of the presentation and name of the presenter should be clearly visible, preferably in a large font. The first slide after introductory slide should include the contents of the presentation Only place main points on the outline slide e.g. use the titles of each slide as main points The contents should be correctly ordered, precise and must not overwhelm the audience. If the purpose of the presentation is learning, the lecture outcomes should be clearly stated (not more than 2-3). Use appropriate action verbs for the making learning objectives.	Use the titles of each slide as main points

Slide Structure	Slides having a good slide structure:
	
	• Display one or two slides per minute of your presentation
	• Write the information in point form, not complete sentences
	• Include no more than 4-5 points per slide
	• Avoid too much *"wordiness"*: use *key words* and *phrases* only
	• Show one point at a time: it will help the audience to concentrate on what you are saying
	    ○ It will prevent audience from reading ahead
	    ○ It will help you keep your presentation focused	

	Slides having a bad slide structure:	The slide will look like this
	• The page contains a lot of words for a presentation slide. • Points are not written in point form which makes it difficult both for your audience to read and for you to present each point • Although there may be exactly the same number of points on this slide as the any good structured slide, it will look much more complicated. • Your audience will spend too much time trying to such paragraph instead of listening to you. • Avoid using distracting animations - do not go overboard with them. You should be consistent with the animation you are using	**Bad slide structure** The page contains a lot of words for a presentation slide. Points are not written in point form which makes it difficult both for your audience to read and for you to present each point. Although there may be exactly the same number of points on this slide as the any good structured slide, it will look much more complicated. Your audience will spend too much time trying to such paragraph instead of listening to you.
Fonts	**Good:** • Use at least an 18-point font • Use different sized fonts for main points and secondary points • Optimum size of font is 24-point, the font size for main point font is 28-point, title font is 36-point • Use a standard font like Times New Roman or Arial fonts • Use a font color that contrasts sharply with the background • Use color to reinforce the logic of your structure • Use color to emphasize a point but only use this occasionally	**Example:** • *Blue font on white background*

	Bad: • If you use a small font, your audience will not be able to read • Capitalize only when necessary: it is difficult to read • Do not use a complicated font color • It is not advisable to use a font color that does not contrast with the background color is hard to read • Using color for decoration is distracting and annoying • Using a different color for each point is unnecessary • Using a different color for secondary points is also unnecessary • Trying to be creative can also be bad	• *Light blue title and dark blue text* Presentation •How to make a good presentation? •Any ideas? Presentation •How to make a good presentation? •Any ideas?	
Backgrounds	• Use backgrounds that are attractive but simple • Use light backgrounds • Use the same background consistently throughout your presentation • Avoid backgrounds that are distracting or difficult to read from.		
Graphs	**Good:** • Use graphs rather than just charts and words • Data in graphs is easier to comprehend & retain • than is raw data • Trends are easier to visualize in graph form • Always title your graphs		

	Bad: • Minor gridlines are unnecessary • Font is too small • Colors are illogical • Title is missing • Shading is distracting	
Spelling and Grammar	**Proof your slides for:** • Spelling mistakes • The use of repeated words • Grammatical errors you might have made • If English is not your first language, please have someone else check your presentation!	
Copyrighting	If you are quoting or using other people's work, images or ideas make sure these are acknowledged	
Conclusion	• Use an effective and strong closing • Your audience is likely to remember your last words • Use a conclusion slide to summarize the main points of your presentation & key points for follow up	For example, return to the learning outcomes
Questions	End your presentation with a simple question slide to: • Invite your audience to ask questions • Provide a visual aid during question period • Avoid ending a presentation abruptly	

Sources:

1. https://www.indeed.com/career-advice/career-development/how-to-prepare-the-presentation
2. https://www.effectivepresentations.com/blog
3. "Improve your communication skills" by Allan Barker – The Sunday Times (2011)

CHAPTER 8

Do's and don'ts during a presentation

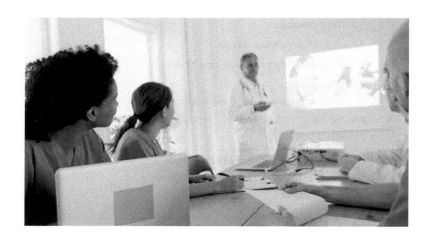

What are most people afraid of?

Recently, a research was conducted in the U.S. when people were asked people about what "their deepest fears" were. There were some interesting results. In order from one to ten, they are:

1. *Speaking to groups (speaking publically)*
2. *Heights*
3. *Insects and bugs*
4. *Financial problems*
5. *Deep water*
6. *Sickness*
7. *Death*
8. *Flying*
9. *Loneliness*
10. *Dogs*

We have already talked in detail about fear of public speaking in the previous chapter. So, we will start this chapter with discussing about things that should happen "during a presentation".

Do's during a presentation:

Put yourself on show

Putting one on display is not an easy thing to do - this is a business of nerves. Being a doctor, you deal with a lot of people daily, and are usually very confident. But what happens when you have to engage in public speaking? Or present a topic in your weekly journal club? Or present ward reports to consultants via PowerPoint? What happens in the minutes and hours before you gather up the courage, start to make your presentation? What is your body's message?

Understand your nervousness biologically:

The nerves, the jittery feeling – is caused by *"epinephrine"* (*adrenaline rush*). Understand this nervous biologically. Epinephrine is released as a hormone from adrenal medulla during sympathetic stimulation and is responsible for producing *fight and flight response*.

Epinephrine causes cutaneous and systemic vasoconstriction which increases blood pressure and produces positive inotropic effect i.e. stimulates the heart and increases the heart rate. Why does it stimulate the heart? To help you cope, to increase blood flow throughout the body and give you extra energy. Extra energy is needed when you are under some threat (fight-or-flight situation). Release of epinephrine is an evolved response to threat.

Epinephrine increases your mental concentration – particularly significant while making a presentation.

So, summing it up, there is nothing wrong with your biology which leads you to be afraid of presenting. The anxiety is probably due to your relationship with the audience than what you have to say. Momentarily, just before you present, there may be some conditions you may find yourself suffering from:

- *Demophobia:* **a fear of people**
- *Laliophobia*: **a fear of speaking**
- *Katagelophobia:* **a fear of ridicule**

There are many symptoms you will need to check for

- ***Rapid pulse***
- ***Shallow breathing***
- ***Muscle spasms in the throat, knees and hands***
- ***Dry mouth***
- ***Cold extremities***
- ***Dilated pupils***
- ***Sweaty palms***
- ***Blurred vision***
- ***Nausea***

It is unfortunate that the audience will forget everything you say. That's the bad news but the good news is that you may not be alone. Every presenter suffers from nerves. The best news is that they also serve some purpose, they are there to help you. They tell you that this presentation matters, you matter. You are the vehicle through which the audience will understand an idea, you are transmitting important information. You should feel nervous and if you do not, then you are not taking the presentation seriously. You are in danger of getting a concentration lapse.

Improving your Communication Skills

The main cause of anxiety related to healthcare is that you put yourself in the "spot" or "limelight" when you present. The pressure of the audience judging your ideas and your evidence, but you as well.

People do not remember reports or spreadsheets easily, but they can retain a lasting impression of a good presentation. If the presenter seems nervous or incompetent, that impression will only stick till the next presentation only. You, the presenter, are at the center of it. You are the heart. Putting themselves in the center of the stage is a quality of an effective communicator. While, an ineffective presenter hides behind notes, slides or computer-generated graphics.

Not everything Is under your control

Nervousness is natural. Once you realize and understand this, it becomes a little easier to handle. "Fear of the unknown" is something that make everyone afraid. There is an element of uncertainty in every presentation, because it's 'live and exclusive' and not a TV you are not responsible for running. Nobody can plan for the uncertainties like audience's mood on the day of the presentation. Nobody can foresee who will be there in the audience and who will not. Any sudden development affecting the explanation or discussion is not under your control. You do not know what question one particular person in the audience will ask, e.g. the brightest medical student in your surgery class may ask a question which you will not be expecting.

This is undoubtedly the greatest strength of the presentations: you being with your audience together, in the same time and place. You are making the information come alive for them.

Transform your fear into positive energy:

During the presentation, the fear should be converted into positive energy.

Use visual aids:

To share the desired information, the speaker uses more visual aids (transparencies, flow charts, images, diagrams, charts, etc.). Each slide should contain limited and important information only.

Face the audience

Try facing the audience, rather than the screen all the time

Organize your visuals:

Organize each and every slide and visual beforehand for presenting in a logical and sound way.

Recognize the body language of the audience:

It gives the speaker the required feedback about the audience if he/she tries to recognize their body language.

Encourage questioning:

The speaker should always encourage more questions from the audience. And he should make sure that he answers them honestly. If anyone from the audience puts forward a biased question, rearticulate it before answering.

Close in style

Always summarize the presentation in the end. Always give your final comments. This leave a positive impression upon the audience.

Be in a presentable in appearance:

To make a good impression, the speaker must have a presentable appearance while giving a presentation. Speakers should always stand with feet far apart to maintain a good balance. Confident gestures should be used as much as possible and use short and simple words.

Maintain audience interest by doing unique things:

Try to catch and maintain audience's interest by using good, positive quotes, sometimes humorous, or any remarkable fact.

Show optimism:

Approach the role of the presenter with an affirmative and optimistic attitude.

State the objectives clearly:

The speaker must write the objectives of the presentation at the beginning of the presentation and make sure to alert the audience about the learning outcomes or objectives of the session.

Power openings for your presentations

It is probably the best idea to start your presentation with an attention-grabber. Greet your audience with a rhetorical question, a statistic that will startle them, or a concept to make them contemplate right away. They will keep engaged or connected with you for the rest of the session. The level of anticipation of each member of the audience should be very dynamic and not taper off. You can make sure that the audience stay connected with you by doing that.

Some Examples:

If you are presenting in your surgery class on how to "suture a wound", here are a few ways you could start your introduction:

"I'll never forget the first time I sutured a wound in the ER. I was so excited but also very worried. I wanted to suture wounds even when I was little, I was a curious child. The patient was a factory worker with a nice clean cut from a sharp metallic sheet. The best kind of wound to begin with. I gave him local anesthesia and he started wincing with pain. I felt all my confidence disappear into thin air. After that, I made as many mistakes as I could. It was a disaster. But in the end, I sutured it perfectly. If today, you are given a chance to suture your first wound today, would you do it? Promise me you will do it better than I did"

Or

"You know what it is like, seeing a perfectly sutured clean linear cut that you have sutured. Truly a work of art. After a long day at the surgical ER, tired and hungry, then you do this. Your first ever suture. That was not done without difficulty though. I lost confidence half-way through it. Today you'll learn how to suture a wound as perfectly as I did, but without making that many mistakes as I did"

Or

"Who among you has ever sutured a wound? Not many I assume? If that's you, you're in the right place to learn it!!!"

Don't these sound much more engaging than

"Hello, my name is Mr.X and today I will be teaching you how to suture a clean, linear wound."

125

Power Closes for your presentation:

we have learnt some ideas about opening your presentations in an impressive way. How about ending your presentation?

Many of us have heard and used the typical lines:

> *"Well, that's all I have for you today. Thank you for being here; let me know if you have any questions."*

And if it's a virtual presentation, the above line is followed by some 30 seconds of awkward waving trying to leave the meeting!

Try these instead:

1. The Bookend Close:

The *"bookend close method"* is used in speech when you need to bring the entire speech *"full circle"*. In this, you will refer back to your original opening or task/challenge. Then you can tell them the important points again. Remember, repetition is the key: if you tell them enough times, they'll have a better chance to memorize it!

2. The Challenge Close:

In the *"challenge close"*, you may challenge your audience to drift off the sideline and take some action. Challenge them to do something amazing. Encourage them to get out of their comfort zone.

3. The Echo Close:

The *"echo close"* is a very effective way to make sure that the audience to remember your presentation. It can also be used in combination with other *"power closes"* options. Build your focus on a *single word or phrase* that will reinforce the call to action. It is recommended to *"create the sound bite"* that continues to resonate in their heads and makes them follow the action plan you want them to follow.

Remember: people will always take with them the *"first impression you leave and the last thing you say"*. The successful execution of power opening & closing should be your biggest priority when creating an excellent presentation!

You should remain calm and relaxed while giving a presentation. And before beginning, wait for a few moments, don't rush and develop an *eye contact* with the audience. Focus on conveying your message efficiently, and use a positive body language.

Create Exciting Presentations

Probably, one of the most difficult things about *public speaking* is *"maintaining the interest of the audience"*. We've talked about engaging your audience previously as well but here we will talk about some more things which you can do to make an engaging presentation, which the audience can enjoy. So, how can you make it interesting?

Sometimes you have to present on a topic that is not exciting and you are faced with the task of presenting that uninteresting content. What can you do is to come up with a "smart" opening to grip your audience's attention: that still is the easy part. How to proceed from there? A clever opening can only take you this far. If you start your presentation strong and it slowly fizzles out, there's a very good chance your listeners will stop paying attention long before you make it to the end.

Keep the audience interested

No matter what the topic of the presentation is, people expect to be entertained when they sit down to hear it, they expect to somehow be entertained. But that does not mean that you need to literally "entertain" them. For example, when we listen to our favorite song or attend a concert or a play, it does not let our mind wander back to things like: any project you need to complete or a piece of furniture you need to repair? No. When you are interested in something and are engaged in it, everything else fades away. Presentation is the art of investing every bit of the audience's attention in what they are seeing and hearing. Watching them interested gives you the much needed energy to proceed.

Use their interest as the motivation to need to go further

The interest of the audience and the undivided attention they give to you, use it as a motivation factor to take the presentation further in the same enthusiastic manner.

Add some excitement every seven minutes

It should kind of, go without saying, an "unwritten rule" and remember this please: no matter how excellent your presentation is, you need to introduce something "exciting" or "big" every 6 or 7 minutes. This makes them surprised, and by surprising them, you'll rejuvenate their interest and their engagement, refresh them. This is known as *"varied stimulation"* in the medical education jargon. This breaks the monotony and catches the drifting attention of some members of the audience.

There are many simple ways to make this happen:

a. In between the slides, display an *image* that is in some way "grand" (large, funny image, but appropriate according to the professional environment)

b. *Ask the audience a question or show them a poll*. Ask an interesting or unique question ("How many people here know which bone in human body is called a "funny bone?")

c. *Change your position* or take a stroll, walk towards or a bit away from audience, or walk through the audience (catches the attention)

d. *Increase or decrease the volume of your voice* in a dramatic fashion

e. *Make a funny observation or say something humorous* – dialogue from a movie, an anecdote, a line from a play, a quote over the internet

f. Do a little "*demonstration*" (involve the audience) – if you are presenting on "Parkinson's Disease", you can show them the pathognomonic features pertaining to the disease, e.g. *festinating gate, mask-like expressionless face, pill-rolling tremors, or the cogwheel and lead-pipe rigidity*

g. Ask the audience to write a *"2-minute paper":* ask them to write something e.g. two points which they remember from this presentation, on a small piece of paper or a sticky note which you can collect later on.

This 6 to 7-minute mark is just a guideline; you can add as many varied stimulations as you like. You can throw more unexpected or funny slides in between your PowerPoint slides. Strike a balance between entertaining your audience and making your message (and your message) memorable.

Choose quality over length of the presentation:

Let us talk about the length of the presentation. Keep in mind that it is the topic and nature of the content of your presentation that will direct how long it will be. Take an example when you are invited as a guest to an event and you are required to deliver a "keynote address", e.g. you have to speak for a bit of time. However, if you are to present a clinic presentation to undergraduates, or your peers in the ward, the quality outweighs the length of the presentation. It is advisable to keep it short, crisp and relevant whenever you can. Pay attention towards keep audience entertained in between too, but do so in as lesser time as possible. Don't compromise the message and let me tell you, the audience will appreciate it. It is easier to hold the audience's attention over a shorter span of time as compared to longer.

Don'ts during your presentation:

Things you should be avoided during your presentation are:

- No slide should be kept on for a longer time
- Being the presenter, don't block the view of the audience
- Don't let the room be too dark. Turn on the room lights else the audience might fall asleep and lose interest in your presentation.
- Don't let your throat run dry, it can affect your speech. Keep a glass of the water with you if you need.

Mistakes during a presentation

1. Body language mistakes during presentation:

About only 10% communication comes from words, 40% comes from voice and 50% comes from body language, according to researches. It is possible that perhaps you have been putting too much effort into thinking what comes out of your mouth and not pay enough attention to your body language?

The body-language mistakes you do not know you may be making

- Interlacing your fingers means you are thinking deeply right now
- Pressing your fingertips is also a sign of thinking
- Blinking more often means you are nervous
- Smiling with only your mouth is a sign that the smile is forced upon or not sincere. A sincere smile can be seen all over the face and is particularly noticeable in the eyes.
- Lowering the head shows makes you appear timid or lacking in confidence.
- Pointing your finger is never advisable. Nobody appreciates someone pointing fingers at own self: it feels aggressive and bossy.
- Folding/crossing your arms: it equated to barricading yourself – putting a barrier between you and your audience – it will make you appear unapproachable, far and closed off and. You should keep arms open and palms up when you speak. It makes you look approachable and communicable.

- Raising your eyebrows: even if it is a sign of being surprised, most of the time, it makes the audience feel that you are uncomfortable.

- Putting your hands on your hips – makes you appear aggressive, depending on how your hands are placed on your hips, but less so if the palms are placed on your back, facing forward.

Body language can be both positive and negative, but the fact of prime importance is that it is greatly *"subconscious"*. Especially when you are nervous, it is less likely that you will pay attention to your body language. You can make awkward movements and gestures that send a message that appears contradictory to your words. (50% of what you *"say"* is with your body!!)

It can be fairly difficult to change your body language since it is largely not under conscious control, it is something you do automatically based on your current feelings. But a good presentation is when the presenter is strong enough to be aware of his body language as he speaks. In fact, a good presenter always practices in such a way that his gestures match his body language, and they both match the words he speaks.

Want to find out what your body language says about you? Make sure you dig out if you are guilty of making any of these classic body language mistakes.

2. <u>Use of filler words during your presentation</u>

We all have noticed people using filler words while they speak during presentation or any other forum of public speaking. And we all know that nobody wants to use them. However, they find their way into our presentations – awful but true. You may know you use them but you keep on ignoring this realization, until they come out in the open and something needs to be done about them.

Filler words – what are these?

"Uh," "um," "like", "ah," "okay", "like"

Small but unpleasant and useless words everyone uses while speaking millions of times. We all have — and we probably don't even realize it. As a society, we are lazy talkers who mostly don't think before we speak, only after it. And till we think about what to say next, we fill up the broken conversations with filler words. They are distracting and do not add anything valuable to our message.

They might not be just one word, but a few words together, e.g. *"you know."* You should learn to stop using these kind of filler words.

Filler Words to Avoid

- You will have to make a conscious effort to avoid speaking those filler words otherwise they will become a part of your conversation without even intending. They make you leave an unfavorable impression, e.g. you are unprepared and don't know what you're talking about.

- Nervousness is a pretty common reason that makes people use filler words. Fear distracts the people and distraction leads them to lose focus. Don't lose focus.

- Getting trained for presentation skills helps eliminate the use of filler words

- Take a pause. Next time you feel that you are using filler words, take a deep breath in. Inhale and use that pause to bring your focus sharply back to your words. The value of saying nothing is often underestimated. Want to refocus? Take a second, take a pause – such an effective tool.

- "There are no small parts, only small actors?" It's pretty much the same for public speaking: There are no bad presentations, only bad presenters. You can win over any audience talking about any subject when you know how to present your material in a way people find engaging. But If you're not willing to put any effort into developing strong presentation skills, it will show in your presentations.

3. <u>Boring monotonous voice:</u>

A lot of presentations are boring because they are monotonous in terms of "tone". Sometimes your presentations need more vocal expressions. In such boring presentations, the speaker drones on far too long with a monotone and flat voice. This lack of vocal expression is very common especially in speakers who do "slide reading" - *read from a prepared text or read their PowerPoint slides.* It is very difficult to have a variable vocal expression while reading.

4. <u>Reading from your notes:</u>

I wish it were simple, then, anyone and everyone would be acing it. Alas. It is not.

It is advisable to deliver a presentation where the speaker speaks directly to the audience as compared to reading from the notes. However, if the speaker's voice is not trained to become expressive, he/she will sound monotonous, flat and boring. Imagine that your voice is an instrument: keep it tuned, its sound will please the audience. You cannot neglect it and make your audience wince.

Importance of voice

Vocal expression of emotion

Vocal expressions are not confined to just the tone of your voice; they constitute a number of other things. It related to the way you deliver and express your words. A good vocal expression conveys emotion and character to listeners, simply by the pitch of your voice, your pronunciation, and your talking speed.

Voice possesses its own personality and its affected by its natural pitch. The reason behind some people sounding more powerful or articulate and others, brash or squeaky is that some people possess a broad range of voice pitch. It allows them to appear incredibly expressive, while others, not so much. Small range of voice pitch leads to monotony. Understand your natural pitch range and work it to your advantage.

Your tone carries emotion in your voice. You can observe how the tone of your voice alters when your emotions are changed: happy, sad, angry, tired or surprised. Tone hold prime importance in making your pitch.

Improving vocal expression

- **Practice breathing techniques: take long deep breaths**
- **Practice speaking slower: practice,** *record*
- **Practice taking a pause**
- **Practice working your pitch range**

How a presenter loses confidence?

Mistakes the presenters make to lose confidence

There is something about speaking in the public that steals confidence from the people. The moment they stand on the stage, in front of a group: their shoulders drop, fidgeting starts – becomes blatantly obvious that *they better be somewhere else right now.* One needs to fight those feelings of "inadequacy" and train to feel and look more confident while speaking.

There are a lot of mistakes speakers make it comes to speaking confidently because they are making five basic mistakes:

1. They Don't Practice

Comfort leads to confidence, and comfort comes from repetition. Each one of your presentations need practice. Do not mislead your mind into believing that you will "ace" it and that it will come naturally to you. It does not. It will not.

2. They Use Passive Language

Sometimes, even after attending the whole presentation of a consultant, you don't feel like you remember anything about what the speaker said. Many medical students complain about that. They certainly had a message but it wasn't clear or decisive: wishy-washy. It's because the presenter did not use powerful language. Rather used lots of "I think" and "I believe", in this way, the ideas appear to be delivered passively. Confident speakers have an authoritative language: they use active words and phrases. Know the difference. Examples of passive voice versus active voice:

Active voice: if a subject performs an action in a sentence, the voice is active e.g. "I perform a laparoscopic cholecystectomy every day"

Passive voice: if the verb acts upon the subject, then it is passive voice e.g. "A laparoscopic cholecystectomy is performed by me every day"

Which type of sentence seems more authoritative and confident to you?

3. They Avoid Eye Contact

"The eyes are windows into the soul"

The eyes are the most important tool of communication. They can clearly express how you feel: happy, afraid, angry, sad, surprised, distracted, or nervous. They can also indicate if you are not confident.

It is via "eye contact" that you connect with the audience and include them into your conversation and grab their attention. The most effective way to include audience into the conversation is eye contact. Avoiding eye contact makes you appear untrustworthy and underconfident.

4. They Don't Use Gestures

A good speaker speaks naturally every time he presents. If this skill is mastered, your boudy movements will be natural. We see people who freeze, fidget or run their fingers through their hair when handed over a microphone, they forget their body movements. Would anyone doing the same would appear authoritative or confident to you?

- Stand up; put your shoulders back, stride across the stage as you speak

- Point toward something really important for drawing audience's attention

- For indicating if something big or small, use your hands to emphasize it.

5. They Don't "Walk the Walk"

A confident speaker believes in himself and his words even if he is doing something as difficult as breaking bad news. He has the content, the data, knowledge of the material and he is well-aware of the words he is speaking. If you're unsure of the topic, how can you be confident speaking and explaining about it? If you've never worked in a pediatric emergency department, how confident would you feel if asked on present on it?

Do's and don'ts during a presentation - conclusion:

Delivering a presentation is a kill which can only be acquired with practice and experience. No one is born a good presenter. In order to become a good presenter, one needs to take care of a lot of things. And make sure that some guidelines are followed and some malpractices are shunned. One of the hardest things about giving a presentation is to be remembered. Use anything out of the above-mentioned things to stay in your audience's memory, forever. Humor is one such thing. Confidence and positive body languages are others. Let these thing help you make your mark.

CHAPTER 9

After your presentation – Reflection and Feedback

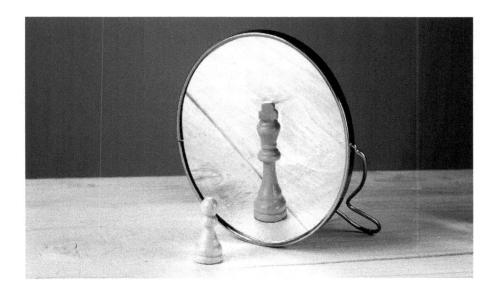

"We don't learn from experiences, we learn from reflecting on the experiences" -
John Dewey

You have done what you were supposed to do. The task has been completed. Presentation is over.

Now what?

Human are the most complex and the most intelligent beings on this planet. That is because they just cannot just *perform* certain actions, they can *review* and *analyze* them later on, *think* about and *assess* them retrospectively: they can **"reflect"** on their actions. Reflection is a little different from assessment and analysis, as others can also do this for a particular person. But the reflection is what is done by the person for his own actions. They do all this as a part of the process of *"self-evaluation"* of their actions and the purpose is to *identify errors* and look for *improvements. How can anyone rectify their mistakes and improve themselves, if they never reflect?*

This "reflection" is really important in self-development. This is because everyone feels threatened if someone else is analyzing their work or actions – critical analysis is never welcomed whole-heartedly. Also, not everyone knows how to give a properly *constructive feedback*, which will also be covered in this chapter. Reflection is the only way where a person can truly analyze himself, free of any judgement of malice. Let us take a look at what reflection is:

Reflection

Reflection is

"any purposeful activity in which a person analyzes his own experiences, or actions/strategy/practice/skills/responses, in order to learn and improve"

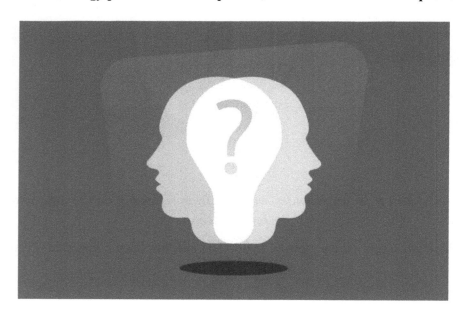

Reflection in academics

It is quite natural to reflect in our lives on a day to day basis. We think about things that have already happened, why they happened, how they happened and whether we dealt with them correctly or could we have handled them in any other way? Better way?

In academia, however, you may be needed to declare your reflections, formally. It is considered to be a part of an overall learning process and formalizing the reflections shows that the learning is indeed taking place. This may include:

a. Reflecting on one's own professional practices

b. Reflecting on one's own academic practices

c. Scrutinizing a professional experience and the way you dealt with it

d. As a part of evaluation of a project or experiment and considerations for improvements in the future

e. Reflecting on already learnt/known things and connecting theory with practice/reality

"It is not sufficient to have an experience in order to learn. Without reflecting on this experience it may quickly be forgotten, or its learning potential lost" (Gibbs, 1988)

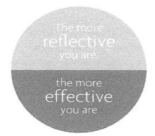

Reflection and feedback, both are very important tools in learning. It is not only important for academics, it holds a very important place when it comes to learn skills like presentations, health communication, patient dealing, public speaking, etc. It is through reflection that we identify our shortcomings and through feedback that we see ourselves with the eyes of the others. Feedback if sincere and constructive, can really add to the process of "self-refection" and become better.

Helping yourself to reflect

Event	***First ever seminar on writing medical literature***
What did I learn?	*I discussed many ideas and that made me aware of many different ways to read, write and analyze any form of medical writing, particularly useful was the article writing. I was surprised by other people's familiarity and expertise in writing medical literature. The ones who impressed me the most were those who started doing that themselves without any formal training.*
What went well?	*I also made some contributions. They were mainly answers to other people's ideas but I was glad I took part and it made me think more elaborately about the whole process of article writing. I also made acquaintances with some editors from well-reputed medical journals*
What could I have done better?	*I could have been braver enough to start writing there in the seminar. I could have started writing the abstract for my article and get it reviewed by someone. Had a preconception that there was a right or wrong way to write an abstract. In future I want to keep my mind open and try to make the most of the occasion.*
Long-term implications?	*Writing an article will be very easy for me now as I know how to approach it now: start from abstract to summarize the whole information into relevant headings. While writing results, it is better to use graphs and charts as compared to plain tables which appear boring. While writing discussion, try to compare your results with previous researches and draw analogies.*

Keeping a reflective learning journal

Keeping a "learning journal" is a very primitive, yet the simplest and efficient way to form a regular and informal. One way of approaching this method is shown below in an example where a doctor wants to become an expert in writing medical literature and he attends a seminar on medical writing and publications. At the end of any seminar, workshop or conference, the organizers and the facilitators always ask for feedback. Most of the times, they also ask the audience to reflect on their learning from that session or whole event.

Reflection after your presentation:

As we have discussed in the previous chapters, the art of presentation is not innate or inborn, rather acquired through hard work, intelligence, eloquence, confidence and preparation. Making reflection a part of the process of learning the art of presentation is a much-needed strategy for not only novices, but experienced presenters as well. Adult learning is a continuous process, it never stops.

As we are familiar with a lot of preparations that go into the process of presenting an excellent presentation, reflection is needed at all steps: before, during and after a presentation.

Models of reflection:

There are several models (methodologies) of reflection related to presentation delivery or any other event of importance. Let us review each one:

1. Reflection before, during and after a presentation:

Let us suppose you have to present a "state-of-the-art" presentation at an international hybrid clinicon (clinical conference) at your healthcare institute. As the conference is being attended by a lot of doctors and paramedical staff in person and also broadcasted live to several locations worldwide, you definitely are nervous. You previously have ample experience in presenting clinical cases and other academic topics for medical students and postgraduate trainees. But the pressure of presenting at this "big" level is making you anxious. The head of the department has chosen you for this and you want to live up to his expectations. You are claiming it as a once in a lifetime opportunity, such early in your career. You are being helped by some peers who are giving you feedback from time to time. Your head of the department has also liked your presentation. You are adamant to prepare well, leaving no stone unturned, however, the most of the day is being spent in "thinking".

The eventful day comes and the presentation happens. You present really well. You are happy with your presentation as well as the response and participation of the audience. Now, you wait for the formal feedback of the audience. Still, being in the midst of all the happenings, you are busy in "thinking".

The overall summarized feedback report reaches you from the quality assurance department, you have done well!!! The head of the department is happy, the dean is delighted and the organizers could not be less proud. The peers are supportive and happy for you. Getting a good feedback doesn't mean that you should not look at the elaborate, individual, anonymous feedback you received from the audience. You start looking at the feedback in detail. You take notes. You start "thinking".

Any good *"learner"* reflects on the learning process before, during and even after the presentation. You can write it down as well. As discussed earlier, in formal academics, reflective writing has a special importance. Writing makes things even more clear.

This method was presented by Schön in 1983.

Before the presentation	During the presentation	After the presentation
What might happen during the presentation? What do you think?	What is happening right now? (make rapid decisions based on this reflection – improvise)	What are the insights immediately after the presentation, and/or sometime later after the presentation when you are emotionally toned done and far from the presentation?
What challenges might be there during the presentation?	Are the thing working out as you had expected?	Think retrospectively, how did it go?
What do you need to know or do in order to be prepared in the best way for my presentation? For this learning experience?	Are you dealing with the challenges efficiently?	Out of all the happenings at the event, what did you particularly give value to and why?
	Think about anything that you should do, say or think to make the presentation a success?	Think about anything you would do a bit differently before or during a similar event in future?
	What are you learning from this experience?	What have you learnt?

Schön's method of reflection (1983)

2. Gibb's reflective cycle:

This method for reflection in learning processes was designed by Graham Gibbs in 1988 to give structure to learning from experiences. He suggested a reflective cycle which included the "feelings" as having an important role:

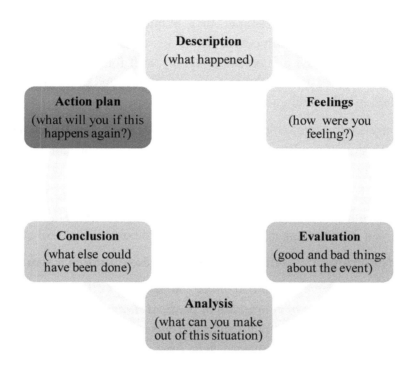

Gibb's reflective cycle (1988)

This reflective cycle offers a framework for reviewing certain learning experiences. Given its cyclic nature, it explains repeated experiences particularly well and allows you to learn and plan from experiences that either went well or didn't. The 6 stages of this reflective cycle are

- **Description** - description of the experience
- **Feelings** – feelings and thoughts about the experience
- **Evaluation** – evaluation of both desired and undesired experiences
- **Analysis** - analysis to comprehend and make sense of the situation
- **Conclusion** – conclusion about what you learned and what you could have done differently

- **Action plan** - how you would tackle with similar experiences in future or any other modification based on your learning experience

Understanding different depths of reflection using Gibb's model

This model works through an experience in an effective way. This can be either be a one-time experience e.g. presenting in a seminar, or a frequently occurring situation e.g. delivering presentations routinely. Gibbs advocated its use in repeated situations initially, however, the stages and principles can be implemented equally well for stand-alone experiences as well. Action plan may be more general in one-time experiences and gives you a fair idea about how it can be applied in your future conclusions.

Stated below are a number of helpful questions that can be asked for each of the stages of the model. It is not required to answer all of them but they can provide ample guidance about what things can be included in that stage, and you may notice that other prompts work better.

1. **Description:** You need to describe the situation in detail here, mainly concerned with helpful questions like "what happened? Where did it happen? What was the outcome? What did you want to happen? Etc.). Feelings and conclusions will come later.

Example of "description" – delivering a group presentation in a seminar:

*"For delivering a presentation in a seminar, me and my colleague was assigned the topic, **"increase in reported cases of depression in medical students with growing screen time."** we decided to divide the presentation into main sections to give the audience good understanding of the whole topic. We decided to take help from recent researches about it published in PubMed. We divided the sections between both of us to make our work easier and stay focused on the content of our sections so that we could do quality work. We also decided that we will start working on it on our own, in our own time. this way we didn't have to schedule time to sit and write it together. At first we expected to sit together and prepare it at work before the deadline (date when we had to submit it for the seminar) but it was getting difficult to find time. After preparing on our own, when we sat down together for final review, it was clear the sections weren't prepared in the same way as we had initially hoped. We therefore had to construct most of the slides again to make them coherent. We had planned to give enough time before the deadline to individually write our sections, however, we did not plan a great deal of time to rewrite if something went wrong. Therefore, we had to work day in and night out, dropping all our important tasks to get this presentation prepared, so that it would be finished in time for the deadline."*

2. **Feelings:** Here, on this step, you can explore any feelings, emotions and thoughts that you had during the experience and how they may have affected the experience. Ask questions like: what were you feeling during the situation? What were you feeling before and after the situation? What do you think other people were feeling about the situation? What do you think about the situation now? etc.

Example of "feelings" – presenting case history of a patient in a group

"Before we assembled and realized we still had a lot of work, undone, I was quite happy and proud that it is smart to have divided the work between us. When we realized that we couldn't present the case well in front of the professor on the bedside, and he asked us to present it again, I got quite frustrated. I was certain that this time, we managed things well and therefore I had little motivation to do it again. Given that we had to cancel other engagements for this, I ended up feeling really frustrated and also guilty for my other clinical batch mate who also had an important assignment pending. This feeling actually helped me to work harder in the evening and get the case presentation prepared faster. Looking back, I'm feeling satisfied that we decided to put in the work."

3. **Evaluation:** Here is an opportunity to evaluate what worked and what didn't work in the situation or at an event. Try to objective and honest. To get the most benefit out of your reflection, focus on both the positive and negative aspects. Never ignore them. Helpful questions can be asked: What was good and bad about the experience? What went well? What didn't go so well? What did you and other people contribute to the situation (positively or negatively)?

Example of "Evaluation" – presenting a research paper in journal club

"There were a lot of good things. Overall, it worked well that I prepared ahead of time and did not get trapped into "last-minute preparations". It is always better to keep things ready. Some small changes had to be made at the last moment, but that does not matter. Moreover, the fact that I had to postpone my weekly grocery trip for an evening of preparation, further motivated me to work harder. That contributed positively to my work ethics. The head of the department and the Dean were really happy with my presentation and use of animations. The thing that clearly didn't work was that when I included a video to be played between the slides, I forgot to check the sound settings. The volume was too low and was not audible to everybody. I even forgot to use subtitles. That video did not add anything to my presentation. I will be careful in the future."

4. **Analysis:** On this step, you will have a chance to comprehend and make sense of what happened. Now you can extract meaning from whatever happened. You want to target the different aspects that went well or poorly and ask yourself why. This is the most important point to involve in academic reflective writings. Some questions that may help you are: Why did things go well? Why things didn't go well? What sense can I make out of it? Which kind of knowledge (e.g. academic literature) can help me understand the situation better?

Example of "Analysis" – lecture presentation for medical students

"I think my approach to divide the topic of endocrine pharmacology of gonadal hormones into two lectures was good. In one lecture, I described the mechanism of action of female and male gonadal hormones, their therapeutic uses and adverse effects. And in the second one, I focused on oral contraceptive preparations, their classification and their three kinds of adverse effects. I think the reason that initial division of work went well was because I could focus on both types of hormonal preparations for different uses. In this way students would not have any difficulty understanding contraceptives. The first lecture helped them to understand the second lecture, although the uses of both are quite different from one another. I have already experienced teaching difficult and boring topics by dividing into sections so students would know aspects of clinical importance. So, I will use my strengths to increases the learning possibilities for my students.

But dividing it into two lectures felt kind dragged or pushed. As both topics were related, some of the information was repeated and students felt that too. I think if I had cut some slides out of my second presentation, that would have helped. I searched through some literature on presentation skills especially in academics where sometimes uninteresting topics are to be taught to students. And I found a lot of books online. I also read a number of educational blogs for this purpose. They really broadened up my vision and provided me with some options".

5. **Conclusions:** In this section of reflective writing, you can draw conclusions about what happened. This is where you summarize whatever you have learning and highlight what modifications need to be made in your methodology that could improve future outcomes. Conclusion is a natural response to the previous sections. Helpful questions to reflect upon are: What did I learn from this situation? What skills do I need to develop for me to handle a situation like this better? What else could I have done?

Example of a "Conclusion" – a presentation gone wrong

"I had to deliver a presentation on needle prick injuries to my surgery departmental staff today. I made a good presentation with introduction to all the needle prick injuries that are faced by us in the department every day, who they can be prevented and further action plan and suggestions were also included. I also included some slides showing the statistics from our hospital about the needle stick injuries and course of action after the injury. However, I forgot that the all the overhead multimedia projectors of our departments were not available for the presentation as the IT department was doing repairs and maintenance work. This just slipped off my mind. I prepared the presentation for multimedia projection and did not make any notes. When I reached the presentation room, it hit me like a bullet. I got nervous that now I would have to present either on the board or verbally: I could remember nothing about the statistics and other things which I had initially planned out. I think I learned a big lesson – never go into a presentation unprepared without notes. Always keep in mind that anything can happen. Always be well-prepared about any kind of situation".

6. <u>**Action plan:**</u> This is the last step where you plan for what you would do differently in a similar situation in the future. It can prove to be extremely helpful to think about how you will compel yourself to act differently next time. You do that in such a way that it will not only be planned, but ensures that you will act differently the next time. Sometimes for people, this simple realization is enough, but at other times, such kind of reminders and reinforcements may work wonders. It can also vary from people to people. Some need constant "push" to force themselves to handle things better in the future. Helpful questions one may ask are: If I had to do the same thing again, what would I do differently? How will I develop the required skills I need? How can I make sure that I can act differently next time?

Example of 'Action Plan' – a co-presenter whose group member always steals the limelight during group presentations

"When I'm working with my group next time, I will try to put forward the concept that everybody should have the opportunity to present different parts of the research during the presentation. I will talk to them about what strengths they have and tell them what I have. Next, if we decide to divide work, I will insist that we give everybody a chance to choose the kind of content they like from the whole topic. It will no longer be acceptable that they always present the important slides regarding methodology and discussion of the research and give the plain results, graphs and charts to me to present. As the audience is not very interested in plain figures and numbers, I feel I have not "shined" as a presenter, yet. I do not feel satisfied.

We all should have uniform opportunity to present every component of research. From now on, I will insist and I will assert."

7. **With the help of independent observers:** This method of reflection is very effective for reflecting on presentation skills. In this method, an independent, unbiased observer can be chosen who sits through the presentation, observes the presentation and then fills a **predesigned presentation "observation form".** The observer can also comment on the deficiencies he/she finds in the structure of the presentation as well as the presentation skills of the presenter, so, in this way the analysis is also being done. how does it help the presenter "reflect"? the presenter also fills a predesigned presentation "**self-assessment form"** – which also in a way provides **"self-analysis".** He can compare and contrast both his self-assessment with the observer's observations. In fact, this method combines reflection (presenter's reflection) and feedback (observer's feedback).

8. **Growth mindset and goal setting:** It is very important for development a truly reflective presenter that he develops the *growth mindset*. Presenters often get demotivated and do not naturally believe that presentation skills can be improved upon. We have all heard them comment that they are "just are not good at presenting." With this mindset, they are willing to accept low confidence, less limelight and ineffective communication – such a mindset takes time to alter. You must focus on these skills in the beginning, but this concept can be taught at any time throughout your journey! Create goals - a new topic, a new presentation skill, a new technology to use, a new kind of animation, a new kind of interaction technique, etc.

9. **Deeper level reflection:** There are many levels of reflection. Some have been described in Gibb's cycle. They are quite similar to those of Blooms Taxonomy, *the lower the question - the deeper the thought*. They are discussed below under "levels of reflection".

10. **Your own model for reflection:** Always take the opportunity to model your learning and reflection whenever possible. After a presentation, model your own reflection, see what mistakes you have made, and record what you have learned from this.

11. **Recorded reflections - reflection vlog:** In this era of technology, create your personal Vlog. After each major presentation or event like conferences/seminars, add to your Vlog. Some upload their videos to YouTube, and others preferred the privacy of simply creating an iMovie or Windows Moviemaker video. With this method of reflection, you will be free to speak about your presentation, public speech; add your slides or add videos and pictures of yourself while presentation. You will find this engaging while allowing you to speak freely about your learning experience. You will feel that you are not bound by

words, grammar, structure, and organization within the reflection, so you will be able to express their truest feelings. You will open up more through this 'on camera' experience, than in any other method of reflection!

12. **Analyze your presentation from the audience's perspective:** Always assess and analyze your presentation using any rubrics (e.g. observation forms). In this way you will understand the rubrics and the typical expectations of the audience from the presenter. Give yourself the same feedback that you believe the audience would give you. Once you get to know yourself and your audience, this feedback can be eerily appropriate! This will help you to see your presenting skills from a new perspective, and will encourage you to make improvements.

13. **Logbook or scrapbook:** It is also an effective reflection technique where you create a logbook/scrapbook for reflection on larger projects and is extremely helpful for group presentations. You can take pictures, define roles, outline responsibilities and contributions. Each group member can showcase their own pictures or share of the group work. Then they can reflect on their roles within the group, the process of collaboration, their impact on the groups success/failures, and on the learning that was derived from the project's completion. Get creative in whatever helps you reflect!!!!

Different depths of reflection

There are many different *depths* of reflection depending on the context you are doing the reflection in and you might want use different **"levels"** of details.

Remember	Understand	Apply	Analyze	Evaluate	Extend

Levels of depths of reflection

Feedback

Feedback can be defined as

"information about reactions to a product, a person's performance of a task, etc. which is used as a basis for improvement" (Oxford dictionary)

Or it can be defined as

"the transmission of evaluative or corrective information about an action, event, or process to the original or controlling source" (Merriam-Webster)

One thing is constant – correction and improvement.

After you deliver a presentation, you should always do two things: reflect and acquire feedback. Feedback is of fundamental importance because only on the basis of feedback, improvements can be made.

In the beginning of the chapter, we discussed why reflection is important. Reflection, no doubt, can help a presenter make an assessment about himself. It gives him a chance to identify his errors and gives him room to contemplate future strategies, which ultimately leads to improvement. Feedback also aims at making things better, but it is a little different because it comes from other people. It is not pleasant to say that neither everyone knows how to give a feedback that *"really helps",* nor it is easy for everyone to accept feedback *"wholeheartedly".* Giving and receiving feedback needs to be learnt. All the principles of affective communication apply to "giving and receiving feedback".

Solely speaking from the perspective of presentations, the audience provides ineffective feedback, most of the times – a feedback that annoys, does not help, criticizes, judges, mocks, confuses and is always vague!! Even if the audience comprises of people of the relevant department or field, it is impossible for most of the members of the audience to give a constructive feedback.

Let us take an example of an institution that organized an annual meeting where a lot of researchers, clinicians and academicians presented their work. A few days after the session, they organized another meeting solely meant for communicating the feedback for that annual meeting. Most of the members provided comments like that were too vague to improve any speaker's performance: *"great session", "good session", "the slides were too complicated,"* without being specific about what made the session "great", "good" or the slides "too complicated." The program directors, however, conveyed information to the presenters that was goal-referenced, tangible, transparent, actionable, specific, personalized. These are the hallmarks of "effective feedback".

What constitutes effective feedback?

We have, and we probably will see people confusing feedback with giving advice, praise, and evaluation. But that is far from being accurate. Effective feedback is something else.

On reviewing the literature on giving effective feedback to new presenters e.g. medical students, house officers, residents or academicians, you will find that the information is greatly outdated. For example, you will find 1980s and 1990s recommendation for employing the *"sandwich" feedback technique*, which involves *saying something positive, then saying what needs to be improved, and then making another positive remark again*. This method, no matter how good, is too long.

Helpful feedback is any information about your presentation that is *"goal-referenced, actionable, specific, and has immediate impact"*. It should be:

- Constructive
- Descriptive
- Nonjudgmental

The trick before starting next comment as feedback to a presentation is to **"self-reflection"**: "How did that go?". This question opens the door to further discussion.

The mnemonic which is helpful to provide better feedback and achieve learning goals is *SMART*: **specific, measurable, achievable, realistic, and timely**, as described:

Specific	• Avoid using ambiguous language e.g. "Your presentation was great". Be specific about what made the presentation "great," like "starting your presentation off with a provocative question grabbed my attention."
Measurable	• Suggest *quantifiable objectives* to fulfil so that there is no ambiguity about what the goals are. for example, "next time, try a summary slide with one or two take-home points for the audience."
Achievable	• The goal of the presentation should be attainable. it should not be something which can not be done or achieved. for example: "Trim your slides to no more than six lines per slide and no more than six words per line; otherwise, you are just reading your slides."
Realistic	• The feedback you give should be relatable to the goal the presenter is trying to achieve. For example, "Relating the research results back to an initial case presentation will solidify the take-home point that for cancer x, treatment y is the best choice."
Timely	• Feedback given directly after completion of the presentation is more effective than feedback provided at a later date

SMART principles of reflection

The ultimate goal of effective feedback is to help the presenter become more adept at presenting his or her research or information in an engaging and concise way, to maintain the audience's attention and ensure that they retain the information presented.

Receiving feedback:

Collecting feedback for your presentation is probably not on your list of priorities or very low on it, especially if you're not particularly fond of public speaking and not making a fool of yourself in front of an audience is your biggest concern. However, some sort of response system should be in place so that your audience can provide you with feedback on your presentation. This is an incredibly useful (also undeniably inexpensive) way to improve your public speaking skills and become an expert and engaging presenter.

Importance of getting feedback for your presentation

Let us consider for a moment that you are a novice presenter and for starters, when people provide you with feedback - even if it's negative—you get a fair idea that they were paying attention to you. They were all ears - listening and watching, and by letting you know what they think about your presentation, they're providing you with the input on your overall message: "from *what* you said to *how* you said it".

That is some really powerful information; it is probably the best way for you to know if the purpose of your presentation is being met. You will know if your presentation is doing what you wanted it to do, whether that is to *inform, teach, persuade, report, motivate or educate* your audience. Who better to share that with you other than the people sitting as your audience?

There are numerous methods to collect feedback on your presentation:

a) <u>Choose The Right Response System</u>

Speakers tend to pass up the opportunity to use *"poll"* with audiences to get their feedback/opinion/response on your presentation or during your presentation, despite it being really useful, quick and easy. It is certain that no speaker wants to feel rejected or be informed of their terrible presentation skills, but wouldn't you prefer to rather know about your presentation if it misses the mark, rather than not knowing? Would you want to continue delivering bad presentations that don't engage audiences?

That is not the only concern. The presentation feedback forces a speaker to self-evaluate. Some will be **overly-critical** while others will be *self-congratulatory* - neither of which are going to help inspire the speaker to improve.

b) <u>Offer a Presentation Feedback Form</u>

Talking about the importance of "connecting" with the audience, the connection doesn't need to end with the presentation. An *"immediate response system"* such as providing your audience with a *feedback form* to fill and return at the end of the presentation is one way to measure your performance. You can also ask the members in the audience to use other methods to provide feedback, i.e. directly to you through *temp email*, on *social media*, or online on *Google or Yelp*. This way, they will not only help you by rating your presentation, but they will bolster your reputation as a presenter with their positive reviews. This will encourage others to work with you. In this way they're staying connected with you beyond the presentation.

There are many other methods to collect online feedback through different applications and software. You can not only collect feedback about your presentations but also create polls, ask questions, take opinions, find out preferences. Two of such easy to use applications are *"Momentive" (previously Survey Monkey)* and *Google Forms.*

For example, you can create a feedback form and ask for different kinds of feedback questions. You can ask for descriptive answers, short one-liners, options, grades, etc. And you can ask for audience opinions. Some sample questions are:

How was today's lecture? Let us know _____

Help us improve _____

Give suggestions _____

What would you like us to talk about in the next session? _____

If you are afraid of the thought of having people *"judge"* your presentation, think about how getting good remarks and positive feedback will make you feel. Also think what will happen if you continue to deliver bad presentations without ever knowing about it!!!! If you are someone who lacks a bit in confidence or tends to be engaged in a high-level *self-critique* of your performance, hearing others give good feedback and call your presentation "inspiring or enjoyable" can go a long way. It will help you overcome your feelings of inadequacy.

How feedback on presentations help you to achieve your goals?

No matter whatever the situation that has brought you to the rostrum — whether as a keynote speaker at conference/seminar or delivering a clinical presentation in a ward — acquiring the feedback for your presentation can be reviving and refreshing. How will you feel when a senior consultant co-worker congratulates you on a job well done? You feel invigorated and motived to continue presenting well, gain confidence and do work that gets recognized.

The same is true of **positive feedback for your presentation**: when you know you've checked the box of connecting with an audience, you are confident and motivated enough to keep making those connections, in an even better way.

Feedback form for your presentation:

So what should your response system or presentation feedback form look like? That is entirely up to you. But no matter how you decide to collect feedback, use the responses and comments to:

- Assess/evaluate what you are doing well and where you need to improve (e.g. increase interaction, increase or decrease talking speed, etc.)

- Understand how your message is being received by others (e.g. repeat your message, interact, inquire, summarize)

- Lead you toward achieving your goals (e.g. increase the performance of your medical students in assessments, decrease the number of needle stick injuries after your presentation, etc.)

Not All Feedback is Bad

The term **'feedback'** has since long been associated with "disagreement" and "judgement", people tend to perceive it as some *"personal attack"*. It earned a bad reputation with some people. The moment they hear it, they run because they're afraid someone will say something negative about them.

Not all feedback is *negative*, not all of it is *positive.* However, it should always be *constructive.* As a public speaker and presenter, you should want to know everything about it. It is the best way to know what your audience is getting from your presentation so you can improve your presentation skills.

Balancing appreciation and criticism – a small guide for giving constructive feedback

We tend to think of feedback as a one-way communication. But actually, whatever is learned from the presenters is give back to them. But it should be ensured that the feedback shows respect for the presenters as humans, as thinkers, even if one disagree with them or didn't learn anything.

- ***The positive feedback should always outweigh the negative.*** Favorable working ratio may be ***five-to-one: five positive remarks for every negative one.*** Sometimes this can be very difficult to achieve! There may not be anything worth learning during the presentation or it may be uninteresting. But it is more likely that you may only be looking at the aspects which seem bad, wrong, incomplete, or inaccurate. Critical thinking does not allow anyone to comment on what they personally like or approve.

- Find positive things and try to focus on them. Praise is a basic managerial and conversational skill - genuine, specific and crisp. Genuine praise does more to help you manage things than anything else, because it brings out the best in people. It helps people to think better and acts as the biggest motivator.

- Make asking this question a habit: ***"What's good about what this person is saying?"*** people should forcefully look for answers and later give those answers to the speaker. If the intention is of constructive criticism, asking these questions will not be difficult. Assume that the speaker is trying to be positive, and give appropriate feedback. You will see that the speaker will be encouraged to be more constructive. Don't try to be much formal with the feedback, it will look like something long, distant and boring. If in doubt whether it is the right time or appropriate place to give feedback, ask:

    i. For permission to give feedback

    ii. How the presenter sees the situation?

    iii. What the presenter identifies as the key issue or problem

Only then should you launch into your own feedback.

- ***Give your positive feedback before any negative feedback.*** Make your own objectives of giving feedback are clear. Explain how the feedback you will give, will attain that objective. It is natural for the feedback to become more positive if it appears ***"forward-looking"***: what you both are trying to achieve and do. The most effective ***negative feedback*** is about whatever is interferes in the progression towards the objective. You can ignore any other ideas you disagree with.

- Be free of judgement. ***Give feedback on ideas and information, rather than on the person***. You should support the comments who you can present evidence for. Focus on the key aspect that needs to be changed most strongly for the better. If you praise them, the presenter will accept the need to change their views or attitude wholeheartedly.

Sources:

1. A short guide to reflective writing (University of Birmingham)
2. Gibbs G (1988). Learning by Doing: A guide to teaching and learning methods. Further Education Unit. Oxford Polytechnic: Oxford.
3. ascopost.com
4. teachwriting.org
5. Improve your communication skills (revised second edition) – Alan Barker
6. effectivepresentations.com/blog/presentation-feedback/

CHAPTER 10

Your professional journey as a powerful communicator and presenter

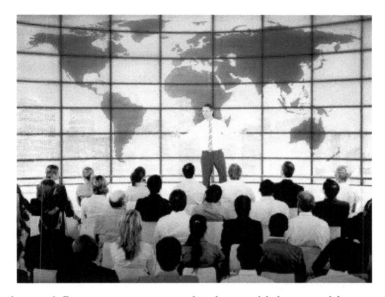

A powerful speaker and fine presenter can make the world dance to his tune. With quick wit, a persuasive voice, and smart twist to his words, he can change a room's point of view.

Think about some of world's greatest (and worst) leaders who have swayed entire nations with their words. Former president of the USA, **John F. Kennedy** convinced people that they could, (later would, indeed) walk on the moon and hoist a flag there. Former prime minister of the UK **Winston Churchill** entreated his fellow countrymen to never **"retreat, fall back, give up" and "fight until the end"**. Former US president **Abraham Lincoln** declared that all men and women deserve freedom.

Words like these in a true sense, transformed entire nations. They inculcated hope in people's hearts and led them to accomplish amazing things. Men and women have entered into battles and won them, just because of words that greatly affected them. Giant companies, businesses and organizations have been built upon merely **"words"**.

While you are a medical professional: a clinician, a researcher, a nurse, a medical academic, or an administrator in a health institute, you may not have anything to do with being a *"world leader"*, you should have a great enthusiasm in improving your communication skills. It can greatly improve your career, your relationships, your personal and professional friendships, and your hunger to achieve your share of *"good"* in the world. Those who communicate effectively achieve great things. They can perform awesome feats: lead board meetings, clarify problems related to health projects, provide solutions to public health issues, perform as an efficient team leader as well as team member and provide outstanding patient care and customer service.

Your professional journey as a powerful communicator begins with steps as simple as a smile on your face while greeting your patients. Your professional journey as a powerful presenter begins as soon as you face your audience even before speaking a word.

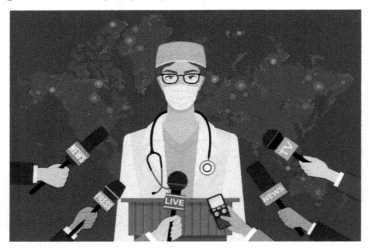

Your professional journey as a powerful communicator and presenter:

Begin your professional journey as a powerful communicator by following these summarized rules:

a) Watch your body language:

People see you first and listen to you later. Therefore, it is not just about what comes out of your mouth, but also about what your body is saying. *Non-verbal* and *non-written* cues are often more expressive and meaningful than what you're actually communicating with your words.

Always maintain *eye-contact*, keep your arms *loose* and *straight*. Try to adopt a *power pose* (if possible, depending on the situation). If you want to express *openness, clarity* and *empathy*, don't cross your arms, rather, keep them *open*. Crossing arms can indicate *disinterest* or *opposition*.

Imagine having to explain a breast cancer patient in considerable distress, about why her right arm may remain swollen after the surgery with *"folded arms!!"*. Would you sound empathetic? No matter what you say will not comfort the patient.

b) Think about your toes

Toes? What do they have to do with your art of professional communication? This may not seem intuitive, rather counterintuitive, but it is actually really smart. An author *Olivia Fox Cabane* is of the view that thinking about your toes *forces your mind to do a full body scan to review, analyze and correct your body language*. She says:

"there's no such thing as too much presence, and presence is always going to improve your charisma immediately. And one of my favorite tools for that is to tell people to focus on the physical sensations in their toes. Like right now, focus on the physical sensation in your toes. And though it may seem slightly quirky it actually is very effective because it forces your brain to sweep your body from head to toe and get you very physically present in the moment."

This may come in handy while presenting a case in front of your consultant and colleagues.

c) Get rid of the conversational crutches

Imagine having to break bad news to a young patient with acute leukemia who was about to get married, visiting you with his family, and you start the conversation with "ummmm.."

Our day-to-day conversations are filled with "watercooler" words like "well…, ummm…, like…, uhhhh… People who are powerful and excellent communicators do not like to rely on conversation crutches. They always have a sharp speech, precise and "to the point" sentences. A simple trick to avoid these unpleasant and dragging words is to speak *slowly* and not just try to fill the silence because when people are not comfortable with silence, they tend to babble.

d) Talk slowly

Many successful and phenomenal actors like Christopher Walken and William Shatner among a thousand others have perfected this trivial but rather extremely valuable tip. In fact, some of the greatest legends of the screen, had faced problems with speech and dialogue delivery. You can use this surefire method and become classics among their peers.

Additionally, we all know people who simply talk a little too fast. It is very difficult to keep up with them, their ideas and opinions. On the other side, communicators who speak slowly and clearly are able to express their ideas more effectively.

A Speaking coach **Geraldine *Barkworth*** says:

"Most of us do speak too fast. A slower pace, using gravitas, is restful and impactful. Listeners have time to absorb your words and if you are speaking to them, you want to create a maximum listening environment for your message to be heard."

You do not need to change your essential self and be something you are not. You just need to pause frequently. Imagine where the commas, colons, dashes, full stops and new paragraphs would begin if your talk was in writing. That's where you pause. Give people time to digest. A pause is like a non-verbal full stop. So take a risk and stop. It is only a matter of seconds or a couple of breaths."

e) Use a "script"

You can have ***post-it notes***, very much like ***addendums***, in your head, for certain difficult and nerve-wrecking conversations (e.g. with a senior consultant, senior nurse, etc.). You can also bring post-it notes to the any meeting to remind yourself of the things you need to discuss or share. You can rehearse this script, again and again, until the important points have been thoroughly ingrained into your speech. *"Repetition"* is the key in order to create a ***muscle memory effect*** between your neural hints and words.

f) Use the "FORD" technique

Meeting new people is always a challenging task in all manners of social landmines. It is particularly daunting for people who do not like to socialize or are introverts. So, people who are less outgoing, thy need to find some common ground when faced with this situation. There is a technique known as the ***FORD*** technique *(Family, Occupation, Recreation and Dreams)* is a good little trick for engaging a stranger.

g) Use the "mirror technique"

Who doesn't like a bit of attention? Some people like to be in the center of attention, they love this feeling. The trick you can use to sound more persuasive and bring your listener's guard down, you should repeat what their words and reflect their mannerisms, quite often. It makes them feel comfortable and open. You can repeat their last statements which shows that you're taking a keen interest in them). This shows care and also clarifies difficult topics, however, it keeps you really busy and almost on your toes. *"So, just so I'm clear, you're going to miss your Sunday match because of knee pain? I will also advise you to rest for a couple of days"*

h) <u>Put away your distractions</u>

Multitasking is a great talent, especially if you are always short on time and you want many things done on time. But multitasking is terrible when it comes to *"conversations"*. There are a few things that make people feel really unimportant if you do not listen to them. For example, if you are talking to someone on your phone, or working on your laptop while trying to maintain a conversation, you'll not find it easy to keep your attention focused.

If you will not stay focused on the conversation, you will miss important parts it. You look disinterested, and there is always a risk that you will lose the respect of the person you're conversing with, e.g. imagine discussing weekend's barbeque plan in front of your patient!!! Keep your phone in your pocket, turn off your computer/laptop, and give 100% of focused attention to that person.

i) <u>Know your audience</u>

Always talk about things your audience may be interested in. Know them. Everything you say should be appropriately tailored to your audience. If you're giving a clinical ward presentation, you can use medical jargon that is common in the workplace. However, if you use the same medical jargon in a community presentation or with junior medical students, you are going to lose people's interest and bore them.

If you are interacting with children, e.g. in pediatrics OPD, kids, if your speech will be animated, it will sound interesting to them. If you are talking to an older adult, phrases that are used for young people might make no sense. Therefore, take time to consider your audience before entering into a conversation with them. *How do they speak? What words do they use? What words should you avoid?*

j) Use the 7 Cs

During any communication, always check these boxes:

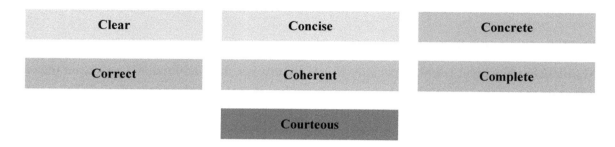

If you stick to these guidelines involving 7 Cs, you will be perceived as persuasive, precise, and compelling. On the contrary, if you are not clear, vague, rambling, use incomplete thoughts, ambiguous and rude, you'll only create problems for yourself and others.

When you are communicating through *writing*, evaluate your piece of writing in the light of the same **7 Cs**. Ask yourself: *"does what I have written check every one of the boxes?"* If not, review and correct.

The benefits of being a powerful communicator in your professional journey

There are no doubts, many benefits of being a powerful communicator. Nothing will go wrong from your end if you will improve your communication skills and exercise your *verbal* and *written dexterity.* Here are a few advantages that come from beefing up in regards to your communication skills.

a) You will prevent situations in which misunderstanding can occur

Not having clarity and strength as a communicator, there will be all sorts of misunderstandings you will have to deal with. And these problems cannot be taken lightly. Such misunderstandings can give rise to grave dangers and problems, both to your personal and professional lives.

By learning to communicate clearly and powerfully, you will definitely improve your professional and private relationships. You will be able to lead people more effectively and deal with problems with more finesse.

b) <u>You will ensure excellence and success in your career</u>

Nobody can build an effective career if they don't know how to communicate well. You will be *a colleague, a team member, "just another doctor or a nurse"*, but you will never be a leader. Leaders not only do their jobs but also negotiate deals, solve complex problems, instill hope, provides proper instructions and advice.

On the other hand, effective communicators will always find themselves leaping over those who cannot. They will always be the ones to get selected for important presentations and cases, picked up to head important projects, and are often promoted more. They are always in the eyes of the others.

c) <u>Your relationships will develop to give you more satisfaction</u>

Powerful communicators who deal with problems involving professional and personal relationships in an effective way and tend to have the most satisfying relationships. You must be thinking why? This is because they can communicate their way out of the problems. Majority of the problems in all kinds of relationship arise from "lack of communication". Such people can let the other people know what they want from them and can also respond well to what other people expect from them. They articulate relational challenges well and interact with people so effectively that the chances of having problems are minimized. They are not only good communicators, they are good "listeners" too because they listen to and understand any opposing point of view.

Those who cannot communicate well will find themselves in hot waters quite often. They will be more frustrated in their relationships and will not be able to work through the problems they encounter.

d) <u>You will prevent unintentional and silly mistakes from happening</u>

You may well have a fair idea how *"words"* can cause problems among people. *Wrong words* or *words spoken in a wrong way* or in *the wrong tone of the voice* can be misleading and hurt someone's feelings and sentiments without any prior intention. Such people either speak too quickly without having a *mind script*, or their words don't *reverberate* (make an impact) because they have no idea about their audience. Thus, misunderstandings will be created which will cause pain to the people involved. One should have a fair idea about speaking *"persuasively"* and have a well balanced approach in verbal communication in order above problems.

Conclusion

Our technologically has advanced, fast-paced world is no place for poor communicators. Those who cannot communicate clearly and effectively, get left behind, both in professional and private lives. Every day, we are firing so many emails, social media posts and updates, text and WhatsApp messages, that there's always the potential for errors. Poor communicators, those who haven't learned the tips illustrated above will make a great many of these mistakes. However, if you invest some time and sharpen your communication skills, it can dramatically set you apart from the crowd.

There is a final lesson that needs to be learned before you place this book on some dusty shelf (hopefully in an accessible location) is related to the *"by-product"* of being a **presenter, academician, curriculum planner, administrator, and communicator**: *POWER.*

Unfortunately, one of the first, and often the most *dangerous* landmine or a booby trap a newer presenter has to deal with, and steer clear of, is the *lure of power*.

As a new presenter starts his journey and prepares for it, his keenness is over the top, unmatched, unbeatable. The whole world seems to be open and welcoming. Expert trainers working with new presenters see the same pattern often repeating itself.

After getting trained and gaining some experience with recognition, the presenters leave with an attitude of *"win-at-all-costs"*: they are enthusiastic, they customize their efforts for every person, go the extra mile and so what it takes without any question or hesitation, they develop a kind and helping behavior.

But gradually it stops. This enthusiasm dies down. When does this desire to help others and work hard stop? When do we begin to get unsure about our own message?

They all successfully cope with the pressures of those initial experiences, but then, a change takes place - *metamorphosis*. After receiving the rewards (praise of participants, peers, audience), begins a belief – our *"professional immortality"*. The belief that we are *"truly talented and powerful!* Surprisingly or not, at the same time, the people who we mentor start to lose their self-belief and lose motivation. They get devoid of the drive we were used to. Or do they really?

This dependence and thirst of power now puts on a ruthless face..

If the novice trainees cannot cope or keep up e.g. they could not prepare a presentation till given deadline, they are admonished lazy and careless. If their slide construction does not meet expectations, they are told that they are failures. This way, they will never learn.

This holds true for senior consultants shunning and ridiculing junior colleagues, particularly junior trainees and house officers. Seniors often "bully" juniors and let them feel unwelcomed and unworthy. When they get transformed as discussed above – they forget that they were also junior and untrained at some point in their careers. All this can lead to hostile workplace relationships. From there on, everything gets disturbed, ranging from *peace of mind to patient care*.

One must always be ready to help others and empathize with them. Sincerity and empathy need to be practiced in all aspects of healthcare, whether it is team work, patient care, mentoring, researching, teaching and administrating. It is mandatory for all the healthcare workers to be ready to guide each other, have no malicious feelings for anybody and must learnt to communicate effectively with everyone.

Having a great communication improves the quality of patient care and workplace environment. And it is the prerequisite for building a genuine and meaningful professional relationships. However, effective communication requires **training, patience and practice**. So, one should not forget to try to study it and train for it.

If you have not yet, start developing your communication skills in healthcare today

Healthcare professionals need to establish, optimize and strengthen their connection with patients. That is the only way to generate the best possible intended outcomes. There should be appropriate communication because both *over-bonding* and *under-communicating* can be regarded as inadequate professionalism. Therefore, effective communication skills in healthcare are essential.

Learning communication and presentation skills in healthcare should be part of your education and profession. Learning such skills makes every kind of job in healthcare, easier and enjoyable. By practicing this, you will get ample chances to bond with patients, your colleagues, other hospital staff, medical students, administration and community, effectively. So, start learning practicing your communication and presentation skills - *NOW !*.

Do it now, because sometimes, "later" becomes "never."

Sources:

1. How to run seminars and workshops presentation: skills for consultants, trainers, and teachers (Third Edition) by Robert L. Jolles

2. mastersincommunications.org/